Listen To Your Body – Decoding It's Warning Signals
By Tony Xhudo M.S., H.N.
Board Certified by A.A.D.P.

Listen To Your Body – Decoding It's Warning Signals
By Tony Xhudo M.S., H.N.
Board Certified by A.A.D.P.
Published by Dawn Xhudo

TABLE OF CONTENTS

Why are we nutritionally deficient

Deficiencies in the US population

Solutions – How to identify the signs of nutritional nutrient deficiency

Physical signs of nutritional deficiencies & common causes of mystery symptoms.

INTRODUCTION

Listen To Your Body: Hello! I'm Talking To You

Hi! This is your body speaking to you, well not really, its just me the author. Often at times our body has ways of warning us of oncoming health problems. Some tell tale sign that may be we can interpret before we wind up in the hospital. How many times have you said, somethings wrong, I don't feel very well, and it hurts right around here or there or I get these pains and start to break out in hives every time I eat this food.

These body signs are about how are bodies communicate various occurrences that may be of a nutritional deficiency or an on coming illness. Many years ago before modern diagnostic techniques, doctors had to rely on our symptoms when ever illness became upon us. They listened to patients heart beats for abnormalities, checked their pulses, the patients tongue, inspected their eyes, skin, urine and even their stools.

Everyday there is some one complaining about a specific ailment somewhere in their body, not realizing that their body is trying to warn them of a health problem. Well, these vital signs and symptoms are happening for a reason, our brain is trying to tell us that there is something wrong going on inside our body's. If every person stopped and listened to what their body was trying to tell them, they probably would have avoided a trip to the hospital.

But, in actuality many people don't really know what to do according to the signs and symptoms their body is giving them. Well, with the help of this book I hope to make it clear to you of how you can basically help to diagnose certain tell tale symptoms your body is giving off, and maybe spare you of an oncoming illness. Our body's have a way of letting us know with specific signs that are really not that hard to determine the possible cause. Whether its by eating certain foods that don't agree with us or just genera aches and pains that come about for no reason, but actually there is a reason.

Just remember, when it pertains to physical abnormalities, there is always a reason for a reaction it gives off. Our body is in constant communication with us, we just need to pay better attention to its messages. Often at times we get complacent and ignore these vital signs with the belief that nothing bad is really happening and it will go a way soon enough, and so we decide to put all those symptoms and signals aside for them to just come back again another time. Hence, when it really gets bad and you wind up in the emergency room that could have been prevented, had you listened when your body was crying out, "hello! I'm in pain and I need some help and looking after, do you hear me?" I've been trying to warn you for a week now!

o, in order to restore the balance we must learn to make that connection with our inner rain and respond accordingly by ***"learning how to recognize the signals by listening to ur body's cries for help."*** By listening and responding to certain signals, like your poop ı the toilet, color and smell of your urine, to the color of your tongue, and the dry spots n your skin, can all tell a tale of whats going inside your body. By paying better tention, you can better prepare yourself for any forth coming health problems that may ɔst you a trip to your family doctor.

xample, when you come down with a headache, you should be able to make a ɔnnection between your behavior, recent consumed food or drink, and your headache. lave you ever asked yourself what might have caused that headache in the first place? ɪid you do anything different the day before? Or maybe drank some wine while eating ɔme cheese?

lave you ever observed, how often you get headaches? Could it be related to what you ːe or drank? Have you ever observed what day of the week you usually get headaches? lave you ever thought that your headache could be of a nutritional deficiency? I bet it ever crossed your mind that there could be a possible nutritional deficiency? Have you ?

ı other words, healthy people are usually healthy rather than sick. But, when a healthy erson does get sick something triggered it in their environment. Become aware of what's iggering your headaches and you should be less likely to get another one in the future. ometimes a deficiency in the ***mineral magnesium and vitamin B2 (riboflavin)*** can ause occurring headaches, or a rise in blood pressure, and even by eating certain foods ke age old cheese that is high in ***tyramine*** a substance that forms from the breakdown of rotein in certain foods. Some people have a sensitivity to tyramine that may increase ɪe blood flow to the brain causing the headaches. ***Other foods rich in tyramine are - rocessed meats, pickles, onions, olives, certain types of beans, raisins, nuts, canned ɔup and red wine. Nitrates and some food colorings are also headache triggers.***

There are many ways to listen to what your body is trying to tell you, using basic tell tale ɔols like your five senses sight, smell, taste, hearing, feel and touch or by periodically, ıeasuring your body weight, waist size, body temperature, and pulse rate are objective /ays of listening to your body. That's how it was done many years ago!

ɪid you know for example, that moderately high cholesterol levels often means that your ody is trying to make more vitamin D with sunshine synthesis in your skin? When you o have symptoms, ask yourself what do they mean. Does it mean that there might be ɔmething more serious that should be investigated? In natural health this is called a ɔnstitutional imbalance . With this book you will learn how to decode these various ymptoms and signals that your body may be giving off in an easy simple procedure that oes not take much time and actually could be fun. By the end of this book, you will ːarn how to spot certain distress signals and avoid yourself or a loved one of seeing the octor and/or a trip to the emergency room.

ı conclusion, learning to answer these challenging body signals and symptoms is part of ealing with the problems of having a good life. Find out what is normal for you, and ːarn to recognize when your body starts to complain. Try and keep in sync with your ody and learn as you go along, keeping a dairy handy can help you list certain foods that you may be allergic to and log the signs and symptoms when they occur.

BIO-CHEMICAL INDIVIDUALITY

Biochemical individuality is the term that denotes we all have different needs nutritionally. Just as our finger prints differ, our outer appearance, personality, we all are unique, but biochemically you are just an individual. However, we do need the same food factors (e.g., proteins, carbs, fats, vitamins, minerals, and fiber. Some of us also may have an unusual high need for one or more specific vitamin or mineral because of our inherited metabolic differences. For example, some us are suited for a vegetable based diet and others are not, and some people can satisfy their nutritional needs by diet alone and others must have nutritional supplements to overcome genetic aberations.

Shakespeare was correct when he wrote - *"One man's meat is another man's poison."* Because of our genetic differences in the way our bodies process foods, most of us are quite deficient in certain nutrients and overloaded in others. Each of us should ask the question, *"Who am I Nutritionally?"* The answer to this question is important for all, but may be especially critical for persons with mental problems.

I am amused by supplement manufacturers who attempt to develop the ideal combination of vitamins and minerals, and amino acids for the general population. This is like a shoe manufacturer trying to determine the ideal shoe size for the whole population.

Because of our nutritional needs, our ability to digest, absorb, and assimilate nutrients varies widely from person to person, and which our organs differ in efficiency for nutritional support. It is rather complex in designing a specific ideal diet that will satisfy every person nutritionally. Biochemical individuality is exactly that, there is no one size that fits all philosophy. But there are some nutritional theories that do recognize differences among certain groups of individuals.

And one of these bases its dietary recommendations on blood types, insisting that those with blood types-A, for example, should eat differently than those who are blood type-O. A great book which explains this in great detail is *"Eat Right For Your Blood Type"* and *"Live Right For Your Blood Type" by Dr. Peter J. D'Adamo.* Both of these books speak a great deal on individualized diet and solution programs for your particular blood type, and how to stay healthy and live a long life. I highly recommend you read them, as you will be amazed on how the four particular blood types evolved in the history of mankind

Basically we all are unique in our own specific nutritional needs and requirements. The best approach is to forget about all the **"should do's" and the "should not's"** you have ever read or heard about nutrition. Instead look for the clues your body provides you with.

3 Easy Steps For Listening To Your Body For Nutritional Needs

When eating, enhance your senses around certain foods. How does the food smell to you? How does it taste? What does the thought of food trigger?

Distinguish the differences between an intuitive understanding of your food and an notional attachment that you have to it. This is important, because food can induce powerful sensory and emotional triggers. Food can induce what is called the "peptide effect", which results in the production of various opioid substances. **Certain foods like wheat & dairy are known for this.**

Follow your intuition and develop a good understanding with knowing what your body needs. In this sense you become more in tuned. Our bodies have a way of revealing our nutritional needs, through the signs and symptoms it will often let you know. **Examples are, white spots on your finger nails signify a mineral deficiency (low zinc levels), stretch marks on skin (also low zinc levels), spontaneous nose bleeds – vitamin-k deficiency & vitamin C, yellow palms – excess beta carotene, bleeding gums- vitamin C deficiency, chapped & cracked lips – vitamin B2 (riboflavin deficiency,** and so on. Every symptom has its nutritional need, and just like every allergy has an antidote. More on that later to be explained.

Your body requires certain amounts of specific nutrients to function well. If it does not get everything it needs, it will let you know in subtle ways. Be the expert of your body, you hold the key to finding optimal health for you. Only you know what feels good and what does not.

Others may be able to observe from the outside, but you are keenly aware what goes on the inside. And if you are not, then its about time you started paying attention. There are also so broader foundational principles that we can apply to almost everyone. For example, a healthy diet can be based on whole foods about nutrition that we can start with. From there you can discover what particular concentration of of each type of food is optimal for you. Some will find that certain foods will trigger negative reactions and must avoid them.

While those same foods may make someone else thrive, hence the saying - "You are what you eat" This also holds true for vitamins and supplementation. We find that some people need to consume a lot more of a particular nutrient to get the same effect that another may get from a much smaller dosage. Two people in the same family may eat the same foods while the other one shows deficient in some nutrients. This is all the result of biochemical individuality and epigenetics.

Bodily Signs of Nutritional Imbalance

Finding your nutritional needs is a process, and are some of the ways to asses your body's responses to nutrition are:

1) Functional **blood chemistry analysis** is an approach to reading blood markers for nutritional deficiencies. But they do not tell the whole story and sometimes can be very misleading. Because, the blood constantly strives to maintain a state of normalcy.

2) Another determining factor that has proved to be a very important and much more thorough guide than blood-analysis in knowing or assessing your biochemical nutritional deficiencies is by a **"Hair Tissue Mineral Analysis Test."** Which by the way will also help uncover any metal toxicities that may have developed through your younger years to

adulthood. You would be astonished what it can reveal and what you may be predispose too, as far as any underlying illnesses go.

(3rd) is a **Urine Test**, but this only measures what the body excretes, and may only be reliable for inf(1) erring the status of chromium, magnesium, and niacin, if their collecte with in a 24 hour period. And besides the content of urine fluctuate throughout he day, depending on the food intake and stress level. **(4)** Is an extensive **Food Intake**

Questionnaire with over a hundred questions for both male and female types that may make over simplifying assumptions. Ignoring the fact that our nutritional needs are not all the. Because, some people may need 100 times more of a given nutrient than whats necessary to sustain life.

Nutritional Symptomatology

Nutritional symptomatology, is when certain changes or symptoms occur in the body when a nutrient becomes deficient. This is considered body language in its simplest form of determining deficiencies or excesses of specific vitamins, minerals, essential fatty acids, proteins, and amino acids. This is a way of interpreting bodily signs to find the underlying cause.

Normally this is done by a computer analysis of health appraisal questionnaires that generate a multi-page print out of what your symptoms are attempting to tell you about your current state of health. It will recommend specific nutrients that can improve your health based on statistical evidence. It is also especially helpful at detecting sub clinical conditions that do not show up on a conventional lab test.

By applying a personal approach, you will be in charge of your own personal health care Your body language will be your own self help tool in determining your possible nutritional causes. This will enable you to take corrective action before your health problems become big problems. It can be used by itself or in addition to other forms of medical or nutritional testing. You can also use this form of nutritional analysis to plan a nutritional program for yourself and also to monitor your progress.

Decoding Your Body's Nutritional Deficiencies

Hands – Cold

Magnesium deficiency, EFA's, B3, vit-E, and iron, (possible hypothyroidism).
Hands numbness in extremities – B1 deficiency, B12 or possible B6 toxicity

Nails

White spots > Mineral deficiency, low zinc & calcium levels.
Ridges > Iron deficiency
Bitten Nails > Mineral deficiency
Cuticle inflammation > Zinc deficiency

Skin

Stretch marks> Zinc deficiency
Dry Skin > Essential fatty acids
Yellow Palms > Excess beta carotene
Rough Skin > Essential fatty acid deficiency
Loose Skin – Poor human growth hormone production

Mouth

Pale Fissured Tongue > Iron deficien
Sore burning tongue > B2 deficiency, B12, zinc > cracked & peeling of lips > B2
Swollen tongue > Food allergy or biotin deficiency
Painful sore tongue > Folic acid deficiency
Gums – Pyorrhea > Co-Q-10 deficiency
Bleeding Gums > Vitamin C deficiency & bioflavanoids
Gum disease > Co-Q10
Pale tongue > low iron

Face

Greasy red scaly skin on face & nose > B2 deficiency
Seborrhoeic dermatitis on nose & forehead > B6 deficiency

Eye Brows

That no longer extend over the corner of the eyes can indicate an under active thyroid.

Eyes

Cataracts > chromium deficiency or excess free radicals
Bags or dark circles around eyes > may indicate iron deficiency, or allergies or food intolerance
Blue eyes and blonde hair > common in hyperactive children > zinc, magnesium, & fatty acid deficiencies.
Blue eyes and premature gray hair > B12 deficiency (feature of pernicious anemia)
Floaters – Vitamin K, vit-C, and bioflavanoids deficiencies
Yellow eyes – Is an indicator of liver problems, specifically jaundice.
Small yellow bumps on the eye lid > indication of high cholesterol deposits.
Bulging eyes and a big lump on the throat – possible Goiter (Graves's disease)

Throat

Thyroid swelling > iodine deficiency, hypothyroidism. And possible thyroiditis.

Teeth

Teeth grinding (bruxism) > your body's stressors showing, lack of vitamin B5 (pantothenic acid), calcium, and magnesium.

Heart

Irregular beat, high blood presure, cardiomegaly > Magnesium & Co-Q10 > sensitivity to caffeine.

Legs

Tender calf muscles > Magnesium deficiency
Brisk knee reflexes > Magnesium deficiency
Poor Leg and Ankle reflexes – this indicates possible low thyroid function.

Note: Some of these nutritional deficiencies that are common and widespread throughout the country that are dependent on environment (poor living conditions/poverty), financial status (low income families having a poor food intake), and poor dietary food choices among average American households, which are **- Copper intake 75%** of diets are deficient in this mineral, **Calcium 40 to 50%, Folic Acid 60% & 100%** in the elderly, **Chromium 90%, Magnesium 75 to 80%, B5 50%, B6 71% in males & 90% in women, 50% in Selenium, Vit-C 50%, vit-D 62%, and Zinc 68%.**

Decoding Your Body's Signs & Symptoms

Bruxism – lack of vitamin B5 , calcium, and magnesium.

Poor Healing – Zinc deficiency and protein intake.

Can't remember dreams – B12 & B6 deficiency.

Sugar Cravings, blood sugar swings, and low blood sugar – chromium deficiency, carb intolerance, and gut fermentation syndrome.

PMS – Magnesium, Zinc, and Essential Fatty Acids

Glandular fever – inadequate liver detoxification mechanisms.

Sensory symptoms – B12, B1, magnesium deficiency.

Mental symptoms – B-complex deficiency, allergies, and toxic stress.

Cervical Dysplsia – B6 and folic acid deficiency.

Measels – Vitamin A.

Muscle Cramps – Magnesium & Potassium.

Shaking hands – Magnesium and B1.

Hypertension – Magnesium.

ensitivity to light – Magnesium.

air Loss – Thyroid, iron levels low, biotin, zinc and essential fatty acids.

requent Colds – Zinc and Vitamin C.

oor sense of smell and taste – Zinc deficiency.

oor Night Vision – Zinc and vitamin A.

ry Eyes – Vitamin A.

arpal tunnel syndrome – B6.

egans – B12 and Hydrochloric acid.

lcoholism – B1 and Magnesium.

ersistent Infections – Vitamin C and Zinc.

asy Bruising on skin – Vitamin C and Bioflavanoids.

amily History of cancer – Selenium deficiency.

ry Hair – Essential fatty acids

remature graying of hair – Copper and B5 deficiency.

Iercury Amalgams in teeth – Selenium and glutathione.

eart Attacks – Vitamin E deficiency and magnesium.

air loss, dandruff, excess ear wax, eczema, excessive thirst, - Essential fatty acid eficiency, biotin, B6, folate, (vitamin A toxicity can also cause this).

kin Tags – Glucose intolerance or reactive insulin levels(may also be a first sign of lood sugar regulation problems).

cne – Zinz, EFA's, Vitamin A, decreased stomach acid, and too many bad fats in diet.

1somnia – Calcium & Magnesium deficiency (possible low levels of melatonin and/or erotonin).

What Your Body Is Trying To Tell You
"Identifying Illness"

inger Length – In a 2008 study in the journal of Arthritis & Rheumatism, it was found 1at women who's index fingers are shorter than their ring fingers tend to have lower levels of estrogen and may be twice as prone to developing arthritis in the knees.

Remedy – Strengthen your legs by exercising and doing knee squats with each leg at a time and stretch the muscles surrounding your knees. Also include more protein and essential fatty acids to help raise your estrogen levels naturally.

Height – According to a study in Proceedings of the National Academy of Sciences, women taller than 5'2" may be missing a gene mutation that helps them reach their 100ᵗ birthday.

Remedy - Quit smoking if you are, and try and lead a anti-aging lifestyle.

Leg Length - Stocky legs may indicate liver problems. A 2008 study published in the Journal of Epidemiology and Community Health, British researchers found that women with legs between 20 and 29 inches tend to have higher levels of four enzymes that indicate liver disease. This could have been the result of a negative childhood nutrition that influenced growth patterns well into their adult hood, says researchers.

Remedy – Avoid exposure to toxins your liver has to process, which will keep your liver healthier longer. Limit or avoid alcohol use and a liver detox cleansing diet would be ideal. Plus use the herb **Milk Thistle** or the **supplement Liv.52.**

Sense of Smell – It was noted in a 2008 study in the Annals of Neurology that older adults who couldn't distinguish the scent of certain fruits, or other items were 5 times more likely to develop Parkinson's disease within 4 years. The researchers believed that the oflactory function may be impacted by Parkinson's disease somewhere between 2 and 7 years prior to diagnosis.

Remedy – Taking fish oil supplements. Omega 3 fatty acids can boost your brains resistance to MPTP, a toxic compound responsible for Parkinson's.

Arm Length – Women with shortest arm were 1 ½ times more likely to develop Alzheimer's disease than those with longer reaches, found a 2008 study in the Journal of Neurology. Nutritional or other deficits during the critical growing years, possibly responsible for shorter arms, may also predispose a person to cognitive decline later in life, says Tufts University researchers.

Remedy – Herbal remedies such as **Ashwaganda**, and compounds like **Phosphitadylserine** have been shown to help prevent Alzheimer's.

Earlobe crease – Multiple studies show that linear wrinkles in one or both lobes may predict future cardiovascular events (heart attack, bypass surgery, or cardiac death.) A crease on one lobe raises the risk by 33%, a crease on both lobes increases it by 77%, even after adjusting for other know risk factors, found a study in The American journal of Medicine. Though experts aren't exactly sure, they suspect a loss of elastic fibers may cause both the crease and the hardening of arteries.

Remedy – Keeping your heart healthy in other ways: like slimming down and loosing a few pounds, and by lowering your cholesterol and blood pressure. Herbal remedies that e beneficial for cardiovascular health are Haawthrone berries.

ra Size – An AD cup may also spell diabetes; women who wore a bra size D or larger
age 20 were 1 ½ times more likely to develop type 2 than those who wore an A or
naller, even after researchers adjusted for obesity, diet, smoking, and family history, in
10 year study published in the Canadian Medical Association Journal. It may be that
e fat tissue in a woman's breast is hormonally sensitive and influences insulin
:sistance, which can lead to diabetes, say researchers.

emedy – Incorporate high-intensity intervals into your exercise routine. High intensity
xercise routines improve the body's ability to metabolize blood sugar by nearly 25%
ter 6 sessions.

'alf size – A 2009 French study in the journal Stroke found that women with small
alves (13 inches or less around) tended to develop more carotid plaques, a known risk
ictor for stroke. The subcutaneous fat in larger calves may pull fatty acids from the
lood stream and store them where they are less of a risk factor, say researchers.

revention & Remedy – Several cups of Green tea a day helps you stay heart healthy. In
study of more than 40,000 Japanese men and women who drank green tea every day
ad the lowest risk of dying of heart disease and stroke.

lood Type – People with blood type A, B, or AB were 44% more likely to develop
ancreatic cancer than those with type O, according to a recent study of 107,503 adults
y researchers at the Dana-Farber Cancer Institute in Boston and Harvard Medical
chool. This may indicate that the gene that determines blood type may also carry a
enetic risk for pancreatic cancer.

temedy – Taking vitamin D supplements of 300 iu or more daily can reduce pancreatic
ancer up to 44%, compared to those who consumed less than 150 iu's daily in a 2006
udy. Fortified low-fat dairy and fish like salmon are the best ways to get vitamin D
om food.

urning Feet Syndrome – A burning and aching feeling of the shins and feet are found
i certain nutritional deficiencies such as vitamin B5 (pantothenic acid). In most people
iis condition becomes worse at night and interferes with sleep. This syndrome is the
:sult of suffering from chronic stress related episodes that deplete pantothenic acid B5
om the adrenal glands.

temedy & Prevention - In an attempt to obtain relief, measures of fanning and
/rapping the feet with wet towels were used. Supplementing the diet with vitamin B5
nd B-Complex with meals will bring relief from this annoying syndrome.

Basic Body Diagnostic Procedures

'ulse Testing – Certain health conditions all have corresponding pulse rates in major
lood vessels throughout the body which can be felt quite easily. Every time your heart
eats there is a corresponding impulse in major blood vessels throughout the body. You
an find a pulse beat in your neck, on either side of your Adam's apple, temples, your

inside ankle bone, and several other places around your body. But the most popular and accessible place to take your pulse is on your wrist just below the base of your thumb.

The pulse beat should be measured at rest with a watch or clock with a easy to see second hand. To check your pulse beat -

Turn one hand palm up and wrap the fingers of your hand around the wrist from the back so that the tips of your fingers are touching the wrist where you are taking the pulse, just below the base of the thumb. Grasp the wrist firmly without squeezing. By grasping with all your fingers, you should feel the throbbing of your pulse beat at once. If you just poke at your wrist with one finger, you may have to move it around a bit before you find a spot where the pulse can be felt distinctly. Do not use your thumb to feel for the pulse. You can often feel a pulse in you thumb so that the pulse on pulse can be confusing, especially when you take the pulse of another person.

Make sure you can feel the beat of the pulse under your finger tips, and as athe second hand of your watch crosses a well defined spot (12-3-6 and 9 are favorite positions), begin to count the pulse beats. If the pulse beats steady and regular, count for just ten seconds and multiply it by by 6. Or count for 15 seconds and multiply it by 4. It isn't really necessary to wait a whole minute to get to your results.

The average normal pulse rates are 72 beats per-minute when in a relaxed state. Athletes and people who exercise regularly and are in good physical condition will often have slow pulse rates, sometimes being 60 or even lower when they are relaxed. Smokers and people in poor physical condition tend to have higher pulse rates. Pulse rates for small children can be normal when more than 90 beats per-minute.

Pulse rates that are above 80 may indicate a health problem with adults. Pulse rates will also increase 5 to 10 beats per minute for every degree of body temperature above what is normal for you. The average normal body temperature is 98.6 F. Normal for you may be a little higher or lower. So if your temperature is hovering around 110.F, your pulse may be as high as 92.

By checking your pulse rate, you can help yourself avoid certain health conditions before it evolves into a major health problem. People with acute illnesses have abnormally fast pulse rates, illnesses like severe anemia, thyroid disorders, and some infections all increase the pulse rate. If your resting pulse rate is regularly over 80 or at the most 85 beats per minute, you should bring this to the attention of your doctor.

Pulse testing can be a great indicator in what your body is trying to tell you and by checking your resting pulse rates and keeping a log handy to frequently record your measurements, you can then help yourself avoid any future health ailments that may arise unknowingly.

Blood Pressure Testing – Purchasing a blood pressure monitoring machine can go along way in helping you take monthly readings of your blood pressure in the prevention of future health related issues. In stead of walking around ticking like a time-bomb never nowing when its going to go off ? They are relatively cheap and easy to work with, and is a great health prevention tool.

holesterol Testing – Another easy test-kit that you can do at home and are available at any drug stores. These kits are a valuable tool to help determine your cholesterol levels the prevention of cardiovascular disease. A great way of establishing and maintainin a orrect dietary protocol for yourself and your family.

igns & Symptoms of a Blocked Artery – With arterial blockage, arms and legs that ay be affected are the more common sites for this to happen. The affected limb will evelop a blanched, white look and will become weaker and weaker because it has lost s blood supply. Compare the affected limb with its opposite, with blockage the affected mb will look whiter in color. If it is affected, check for a pulse at the ankle or on top of e foot. You will not be able to feel a pulse if there is blockage there. If so, seek medical elp immediately!

hyroid Test – There are many people that have thyroid issues that are causing them so any health problems, so of them are not even aware its there thyroid that is causing ese problems. With a simple home thyroid test that you can do with a basal ermometer can help you to determine of its malfunction.

our thyroid sits just below your Adam's apple and it's wings are on both sides of your achea. To test quickly, run your fingers gently along the sides of your throat where your yroid sits and see if there are bumps or swelling. If you feel any swelling around this rea, then you need to explore this even further with a basal temperature thermometer.

his test is easy to do and is surprisingly accurate. Purchase a basal thermometer at your rug store (this is different from the oral one) every morning before you get up out of ed, place the thermometer under your arm pit for 5 to 10 minutes. Record the reading or 3 to 4 days, your normal temperature should be 97.8 and 98.2 on the average. If its is ot, then you may want to test it further with the help of your doctor and ask your a pecific complete thyroid panel test.

igns & Symptoms of Low Thyroid – are cold hands and feet, difficulty in swallowing ills, hair loss, digestive disturbances, emotional issues for no apparent cause, lack of nergy, susceptibility to colds and infections, puffy eyes, inability to lose weight, and ore.

emedy – Herbal remedies are quite helpful in restoring under active thyroid problems – erbs such as Ashwaganda, Kelp(iodine), the amino acid Tyrosine, and glandular extracts f thyroid all seem to help quite effectively.

drenal Gland Test – If you are experiencing more than your normal amounts of stress, ere are simple home tests that you can do to check the health of your stress glands to elp determine adrenal fatigue. With a simple home blood pressure test machine sphygmomanometer) sold at drug stores, you can check your blood pressure by first king it in a lying position, resting for about 5 minutes and then again in a standing osition.

Normally in people with low functioning adrenal glands or hypo-adrenia, their blood pressure will be low to begin with. By taking the two different readings, lying and standing and measuring the difference between the two and the pressure drops in the standing position by 10mmhg's or more when you stand up. You more than likely have weak adrenal glands that should be corrected. You can also perform a **"Adrenal Salivary Test"** that can be purchased as well through the internet websites, this test is also a great indicator of adrenal gland functioning.

Signs & Symptoms of Weak Adrenal Glands – Are inability to handle stressful conditions, weak and tired feeling, obesity, low blood pressure, burning leg syndrome, low thyroid levels, dizziness standing up quickly from a seated position, and more. This can be a serious condition that should be taking care of immediately, see your doctor.

Remedy – High protein foods and complex carbohydrates help to provide the adrenal glands with all the necessary nutrients it needs to restore health and activity to these vital glands. Supplements like B-Complex, especially B5 and vitamin C both help to support the production of adrenal gland hormones.

Our body can speak volumes about what ails it, from all the various warning signs and symptoms that it can give off. Learning how to tell and decode these vital signs is the key in preventing ailments and illnesses from manifesting. Some of these signs are harmless and some are early warning signs that we should pay attention to before it becomes too late. With many of the procedures listed in this book , you will be able to help yourself become more aware of possible health related problems.

Preventive Medicine

Today, we have so many available home self test-kits that can enable us to quickly diagnose simple health related issues that can become more serious if left untreated. And with the major changes to the nations health care system looming, it may be more important than ever for you to keep track of your own physical health. By emphasizing preventive care you can head off illness before it becomes too serious.

Some of the more worrisome body signs are already well known, like **breast cancer** that affects women and knowing how to check regularly for breast lumps, dimples, swelling and discharge that can signify cancer, and to have regular mammograms done. **Excess belly fat** is also becoming a notorious body sign as well and could be a heightened risk of diabetes, high blood pressure, stroke, heart disease, gall bladder disease and possible cancer. Waist to hip ratios are especially telling; If a man's waist is larger than his hips, or a women's waist is more than four-fifths her hip circumference, that's a sign that dangerous visceral fat is surrounding an abdominal organ. Evaluating skin cancer has also gotten significant publicity. Learn to evaluate spots on your skin that may be a sign of skin cancer.

Asymmmetrical shapes, or a **jagged** and **irregular border** or suspicious **color** and **diameter** larger than a pencil eraser that may be elevated and even all distinguish possible skin cancer. Regular check ups on your skin should be considered and observed, especially if you use tanning beds or sun bath excessively.

ther possible signs of illness that can be distinguished with body signs and symptoms e thyroid disease, a common problem with so many women today. Obvious signs for w thyroid that can manifest are – loss of hair, slow growing hair, dry and brittle hair, ittle finger nails, easy weight gain, cold extremities hands and feet, swollen neck pecially around the Adam's apple, and poor reflexes.

nger nails can tell tales as well, white nail beds – the skin under neath the nail – can gnify anemia. Nails that are white near the cuticles and red and brown near the tip can e a sign of kidney disease. Irregular shaped brown or blue spots in the nail bed can be elanomas. Finger tips that are blue or clubbed can be a sign of lung disease and nerally there would be more significant signs as well.

any of these same signs occur on the toe nails as well. But the feet can be critical for her reasons too. Feet can tell you a huge difference about health and circulation, says r. Denman, the Duke nursing instructor. Feet are the first place that vascular disease can low up where the blood vessels are the smallest and the farthest away from the heart. irculatory problems, like numbness and tingling in the feet, like peripheral neuropathy, damage to the nerves that often begins at the extremities. Both are signs of ncontrolled diabetes. Thats why people with diabetes are urged to check their feet every y for any kind of scratch or lesion.

eeth are another open window into overall health. The New York University's College f Dentistry and the College of Nursing have checked patients at the university's free ental clinic for other health issues. And more than 60% of the patients referred from the inic met the criteria for hypertension, and 30% of them had diabetes or pre-diabetes.

rarer cases, gums can bleed and become inflamed from leukemia. Bulimia can also ave tell tale acid marks on the back of the teeth and missing teeth can be a sign of poor utrition, advanced gum disease or long term drug use. Some other interesting body signs ke short leg length has been linked to a higher risk for diabetes, atherosclerosis and eart disease, which can all be due to poor nutrition in utero or early childhood. Several ther studies have found that the shorter a man's index finger in relation to his ring finger, e more aggressive he's likely to be due to a higher testosterone level.

s you can see there are many vital tell tale signs that our bodies can give, and being igilant about your body signs can help you prevent ill related consequences that you on't necessarily have to suffer. Prevention and observation are the keys here, learn and udy some of these vital signs and make up a list if any apply to you, and help yourself revent any unnecessary problems that can occur by taking the corrective measures.

How To Decode Your Basic Body Language
and Decode What People Really Think

he latest research indicates that there are well over 70% of our communication is done on-verbally. Often times the body can speak louder than words. People have a way of xpressing their feelings, emotions, attitudes and intentions through auspicious signals arough the way they were their clothes, body movements, and certain particular estures that they often tend to give off. Some examples of body gestures when people are <u>**lying**</u> are:

1. Covering of the mouth with your hand.
2. The Nose touch – scratching and itching
3. The eye rub
4. the ear grab
5. the neck scratching
6. the collar grab
7. fingers in the mouth

Gestures of **procrastination and boredom** that people will often exhibit are :
1. Hand to chin gesture
2. Yawning
3. Chin stroking
4. Head rubbing

Body language signs is like listening to some one talk if you know how to read it. **The eyes,** called the window of the soul express and reveal what the person really feels by the intensity and direction of their stare can reflect a person's thoughts, here are some different scenarios:

- **Staring hard without interruption accompanied b small pupils could mean an invasive threat.**
- **Gazing up and down > is an appraisal of sexual attraction (this usually accompanies both men & women) although women are usually more discreet.**
- **Glazing sideways intermittently but repetitively usually shows concern and nervousness.**
- **An avoiding gaze > could show feelings of guilt, lying, or being just uncomfortable about the subject at hand.**
- **Gazing regularly and direct when face to face > shows a positive attitude and interest in you and the subject at hand.**
- **Blinking Prolonged > means losing interest, which is normally accompanied by a raised eye brow.**
- **Excessive blinking > shows romantic interest (if pupils are dilated) and can also mean a sign of stress, or lying about something.**
- **Rolling the eyes upwards > shows disagreement or exasperation if its very obvious.**

Learning how to read body signals and language can help you determine what people ar thinking about. Whether it may be something their lying about, their interest, or other possible tell tale signs. A **smile** is another way of interpreting certain signals, like happiness, friendly attitude, interest, and hate.

- **A forced smile > can be usually out of politeness. It also can mean the person is not telling the truth. Research also does indicate that a larg majority of people unconsciously recognize the sincerity of your forced smile simply by looking at the top half of your face.**

- A Closed smile > can mean that they are trying to be polite, or they are embarrassed by their teeth.
- A whole face smile > is a genuine smile indicating happiness, honesty and openness to communication.
- Covering of the mouth smile > could mean they are lying or just unconfortable about he situation.

he **lips** too can give off various indications of frequent gestures of importance, here are few samples:

- Puckered lips > tasted something sour or their just recalling a similar feeling.
- Pursed lips > indicates worry and disapproval.
- Lip biting > shows nervous habits, anger and anxiety.
- Lip licking > sexual interest.
- Looking at your Lips > unconsciously assessing the pleasure it would be to kiss your lips, and a romantic interest in you.

he **head and hair** can also show obvious signs of body language, some samples are:

- Twirling hair around with your fingers > shows in women nervousness and anxiety.
- Touching the hair > especially women, can show flirting clues of romantic interest.
- Keeping a level head > shows a relaxed demeanor, self assurance and confidence.
- Tilted head > shows they are paying attention to you when talking.
- Nodding of the head > reflects agreement in most parts of the world, and a genuine interest.

he **Hands** are another body signal that have interesting clues of behavior, examples are:

- Hiding their Hands > means being secretive, not inclined to communicate, and could be possibly lying.
- Touch your face while kissing > shows a genuine romantic interest, also a slow seduction process.
- Hands in their pockets with thumbs out > shows confidence and feeling superior.
- Handshakes Palms facing down > shows domination.
- Bone crunching hand shake > shows enthusiasm, domination.
- Limp handshake > does not like being touched or is submissive.
- Double handshake > indicates a mini embrace, or is very friendly and an invitation to being trusted.
- Hands in front of he groin or chest area > a closed pose, protective, defensive and not at ease.

Note: If you are trying to influence someone or trying to seduce a man or a women, subtly use the double handshake and briefly brush the back of their hands to effectively create a double handshake for a split second. At an unconscious level, this creates a muc[h] stronger bond between you and the other person, research shows that it makes the perso[n] trust you and like you more.

People unknowingly give off amazing clues to what their really trying to tell you. Most of these body language signals or clues were studied by FBI when profiling certain individuals in studying particular individuality types. Amazingly so many of these gestures hold to be true due to many experimentation's done on hundreds of individuals.

Here are some examples of what the **arms and legs** can tell:

- **Arms by the side and away from the body > means confident, strong.**
- **Closed or crossed > means uninviting and protective.**
- **Touching someone's arms > sympathy, or a subtle invitation to trust or intimacy.**

Note: Just by touching someone's hands or arms makes them more likely to trust you an[d] like you. You can use this method to influence someone.

Leg samples of body language are :

- **Swagger (men), or discreet swishing of the hip walk (women) > indicates seductive, subtle flirting.**
- **Crossed over the knee or ankle > means your relaxed, but not completely at ease.**
- **Ankle crossing over the knee > (mainly men) > shows confidence, arrogance or assertiveness.**
- **Leg twining > (women) shows a physical attraction.**
- **Uncrossed legs, slightly open > is an inviting body language open to communication.**
- **Touching their thighs > an unconscious sign of attraction.**

The **Feet** in a nutshell, point in the direction our minds want to go, interesting examples are:

- **Jiggling or tapping > nervous gesture, bored.**
- **Turned in your direction > indicates an interest in you.**
- **Feet pointing towards the door > shows a lack of interest in you, and inpatients. Avoid this position if you are trying to influence someone.**

The **Face, Ears, Chin, Adam's apple, and the Nose** can express strong body language indications, here are some interesting samples that will help you decoding these signals:

- **Scratching of the ears > indicates a lack of confidence, and could also be a sign of deceit, and usually with this the ears get redder.**
- **The Chin resting in the hand gesture > means possibly bored, faked interest.**

- ↟ **Rubbing with the forefinger** > might not believe what they are being told.
- ↟ **Stroking the chin** > means interested, paying attention during the conversation, and if they are silent they are pensive.
- ↟ **A jumping Adam's apple (men)** > shows anxiety, embarrassment, and stress.
- ↟ **Touching your nose when talking** > might be trying to hide something.
- ↟ **Nose flare** > indicates agitation, anger.
- ↟ **Nose twisting to one side** >means disagree or dislike.
- ↟ **Nose wrinkle**> indicates repulsion.

Important Signs Your Poop & Pee Is Trying To Tell You
"You Shouldn't Try To Ignore"

How many people normally go into the bathroom to go about their business in relieving themselves, but always fail in examining their body's excretions ? Have you ever wondered what is considered normal or you were to embarrassed to ask? Or have you ever wondered why sometimes poop and urine can smell very awful? Well, analyzing your poop can be a quick way of determining health problems. A healthy bowl elimination time is between 16 to 24 hrs from eating to eliminating, yet the average American takes 96 hrs – that's 4 days of rotting waste product stuck in your colon and oozing out into your bloodstream!   The average American colon carries 5lbs of putrid, partially-digested meat in their colon and another 5 to 10lbs of fecal matter that has been packed with mucus for years to form a hard lining in deformed folds of the colon.

Is it any wonder you may suffer from health problems like – fatigue, bad breath, irregular bowls, skin outbreaks, unexplained pain, embarrassing and smelly gas, and more! And when your colon is clogged – it will do anything to send out an S.O.S. for health! That means giving you "dragon breath" and B.O.! A strong body odor, especially under your armpits.

Here are some interesting facts about your poop and pee. Food that we eat actually has to travel through about 30 feet of intestines before it actually comes out. The average human will produce about 9,000lbs of poop over the course of his or her lifetime. And the clue to disease may just be sitting in your toilet bowl. So, make sure before you flush to analyze this valuable information. Here are some clues:

Little lumps > indicates that food is staying in the intestines too long and water is being reabsorbed, also possible sign of poor liver function, and lack of exercise. A lack of dietary fiber can also lead to these hard little pellets.

Too liquidy > Food is moving through the intestines too quickly, so water is not being absorbed, due to an increase in fiber, a cleanse, or an infection.

Pencil thin poop > A mass in the colon could be constricting the stool. It may be an indicator of colon cancer.

Floats & smells > body is not properly absorbing fats. It could also be the result of a malabsorption condition, weight loss, drugs, or Olestra.

Hard & dry > Food is staying in the intestine too long, so water is being reabsorbed. This could be due to dehydration, constipation, and medications.

Non-existent Poop > if you're not going at all, your constipated! Drink plenty more water and increase your fiber intake.

Green poop > food is going through your digestive system faster than normal resulting in bile not being able to change color from green to brown. You may also see this in diarrhea. If your have green feces on a regular basis, it could mean a bigger problem. Check with your family physician. Detoxifying may be a good solution here. Also note that eating an abundance of green leafy vegetables containing chlorophyl can cause this as well. Celiac disease may also cause green poop, as well as Chrohn's disease and an Ulcerative Cholitis as well as Irritable Bowl syndrome.

Yellow-colored poop > indicates your food is moving too quickly through your intestines. If poop is greasy or foul smelling, it may indicate excess fat caused by malabsorption of nutrients.

Gray or ashy colored poop > indicates undigested fats or heavy use of prescription drugs or over the counter remedies that contain aluminum hydroxide. It can also mean a lack of bile in the stool that may be caused by inefficient bile duct function.

Black poop > is a sign blood is present in the stool, and you could be experiencing less than optimal health in the upper gastrointestinal tract.

Bright Red poop > Indicates fresh bleeding. Distended rectal veins may also be the source of bleeding.

The bottom line : A normal bowel movement happens every 60 seconds of sitting on the toilet. There should be no straining, discomfort, bleeding, or foul odor accompanied with your bowel movements. And wiping afterwards should be easy and simple – using one o two sheets of toilet paper!

A colon cleanse may be beneficial, and you should talk with your family doctor if you notice any changes out of which is normal as it could be an indication of something more worse. In the meantime, eat whole foods rich in fiber such as raw vegetables that contain soluble and insoluble fibers which can help promote a healthy digestive system. Drink plenty of water, the more fiber you eat the more water you need to drink. Water is an excellent way to flush out impurities and toxins from your intestinal tract. Exercising more regularly works wonders if you need help with constipation. Take care of your colon and it will take care you. When you do – your body can properly absorb nutrients to fuel every cell in your body!

Urine Problems & Indications

The average adult bladder holds 16oz. And one often feels the urge to empty their bladder around 8oz. If you feel burning while urinating it could mean a possible infection, or if you see blood in your urine please see your doctor immediately. **Here are**

me of the signs of urine problems:

- **Pale pee** > means your drinking lots of water or liquids.
- **Dark Pee** > is a sign of not drinking enough water, and could also be the sign of possible kidney problems.
- **Low pH** > or acid urine > could result from lung disease, diabetes, or starvation.
- **High pH** > or a high alkaline urine, could mean a sign of kidney disease or infection.
- **Bright Yellow Pee** > this is a result of B vitamins and beta carotene.
- **Murky Pee** > could be the symptoms of a UTI or possible kidney stones.
- **Red or Pink Urine** > could indicate the presence of blood which is a sign of a serious problem.
- **Foamy Urine** > result of a large amount of protein in your diet.
- **Orange Urine** > can be caused from eating black berries, rhurbarb, or medication. Could also indicate jaundice or dehydration.
- **Green or Blue Urine** > could be the result of something you ate, be it asparagus, or something with a blue dye, or certain medications or supplements.
- **A sweet smelling odor** > could be a sign of possible diabetes.

nce medieval times doctors used urine to diagnose diabetes. The sheer volume of quid, the dark color, frequent urination, and a sweet taste were both tell tale signs. And ey knew that an infection makes pee cloudy and smell bad. A bladder-kidney infection ith a strong smell, pain on urination with a pinkish or red color, could indicate a adder, or even a kidney infection is taking place.

idney stones, the urine would appear very **cloudy or murky** from the calcium in the ones that washes into the urine. And high calcium levels sometimes called blue diaper children because the urine can turn blue from the presence of calcium. This usually erts to a condition called hypercalcemia, or too much calcium.

len over 50 tend to show up blood in the urine from an enlarges prostate gland and from erhaps passing a kidney or a bladder stone. Women also tend to get more bladder fections especially as they approach menopause. Very heavy, darkish, burning urine, at can have blood in it, is almost always a warning sign of infection.

emember, most urine color changes are not something you need to be concerned about nd are a variation of how your urine filters throughout the day. However, if you can not etermine that your urine color changes from medications, vitamins, foods, water intake, r if you have the warning signs listed here, please see your doctor immediately.

our body is a magnificent machine, functioning 24/7 every day of your life. When lings go awry, it generally does not shut down without warning, like a light bulb that urns out without warning. Instead it sends us little signals or lets say biological taps on le shoulder trying to let us know that something is a miss. How often do we stop and lke the time to see or analyze what may be wrong ?

Physical signs and symptoms are ways that your body tries to alert you that something needs to be attended to. You can do so much by just taking the time and the initiative to try and decipher the signs and symptoms to get to the cause of the problem, and not to just suppress the end result of ill health. Interpreting these little quirky Morse codes doe not really require a deep level of body awareness. With the help of this book, you can gain an advantage in taking the time to decipher and identify most common health conditions, before they manifest into some thing more serious.

When you listen long and hard enough to your body, you will begin to differentiate sensations and feelings. Your body will not lead you astray if you know what it needs and respond to it appropriately. We rarely listen to our bodies and then pay the price late for being so naïve, But instead rush to our doctors office to explain the symptoms we were receiving. And how many times have you injured yourself, after claiming that you can see it coming? How many times have you made yourself sick, after saying that you know how to listen to your body? I guess the lesson is always learned afterwards, but it does not have to be that way. Learning to listen to your body, respond to its every signal and be in sync with it – that's something that can be done without so much effort.

How To Listen To Your Body – Form A Habit

Habit builds excellence throughout the many aspects of life. Listening to your body through an act of habit can be an easy task, so learn to react to signals your body is sending, that you've ignored most of the time. The body speaks volumes of what ails it, so be vigilant for anything new or unusual about your body. The more engaged you can be in learning its symptoms and signs, the better you will become.

Awareness is the link, every cell of your body knows when you are not happy, anxious o stressed. A cell's awareness is expressed in chemical reactions instead of words and the message comes through loud and clear, make no mistake. The most basic elements of listening to your body are – feel what you feel, accept what you feel, be open to your body, trust your body, and enjoy what your body wants to do. These are all primary things to pay attention to, Keep your attention on sensations until they disappear. Every answer to every question you have about your health will ultimately be answered throug the process of observing your body!

If we are able to listen to our body's, being over weight and a lot of other physical problems would disappear. Heart attack victims often slip into a denial syndrome and sa things like, "It's only heartburn", "It will go a way in a few minutes", etc. And how man cancer victims were too busy to have that enlarged mole looked at? Or when you were enjoying that glass of wine, and your body is telling you that one glass is enough, but your mind reaches out for another glass.

We all get too insensitive to our bodies messages and don't go for medical help when we should. The grave yards are filled with people that didn't listen to their bodies. Illnesses and disease always manifests slowly, and this is when one needs to first start paying attention to the signs and symptoms. No one knows your body better than you do, make habit of listing certain clues and signs when you first start to notice that something migh be wrong. Notice if the symptom your receiving might be a nutritional deficiency that an be regulated and restored, or if its some thing more serious, learn to tell the difference of signs and symptoms of a more serious nature.

For example, how does your body feel right now? Lets go a head and take a simple inventory. From the head to the toes, what's going on at the present moment? How's your head feel ? Are you depressed, stressed, happy or sad? How's your neck, your back? How's your stomach doing? How about your muscles? Your energy levels? Are you tired or sleepy? Good or bad, what signals you are getting? Beyond the here and now, what's your body trying to tell you lately? Any changes since the beginning of this challenge? And most importantly are you accustomed to listening to what your body has to say?

Everything about our culture, seems to discourage us from doing just that. From the commercials insisting we don't need to put up with that headache, so we'll just pop a couple of aspirins. That's exactly what most people do, and taking a body hint isn't exactly on the top of most people's priorities. Or that indigestion we get from eating that second slice of pizza, so we'll try some Pepcid AC.

It is amazing how people just don't stop and listen to what their body is trying to tell them. They knowingly ignore pain, discomfort, low energy levels, go to work sick as a dog and eat a diet for much of their lifetime that leaves them sluggish and over weight. It's only when serious illness strikes that they take up notice, and ironically sometimes serious illness teaches us to listen to our bodies, to discover how symptoms – however subtle they can be, as a crucial barometer for larger issues. Therefore we'll do well to heed its warnings and clues before it smacks us right over the head with a club.

Too often, we tend to surrender the power that comes from reading and knowing our bodies, only to relinquish it to doctors and other practitioners, either because we genuinely believe theirs is the only substantive opinion or because we don't really want to take responsibility for our own health. Learn to appreciate your own ability to listen to your body's signals and follow through with it.

Also, take advantage of modern technology and learn from self-assessment, as a glucose monitor can be a handy tool. A heart rate monitor is a good device to have also. A note book and pen might be also a good idea. So by all means, take advantage of technology and use it to help hone your own perception of listening to your body talk. Think for a moment, about all the sensations that your body can produce -

- **⅄** **Positive and negative feelings, fatigue, foggy thinking, and dizziness.**
- **⅄** **Digestive disturbances or issues, rapid heart beats and breathing.**
- **⅄** **Back pain, achiness, stiffness, neck tension, headaches and migraines.**
- **⅄** **Stuffy nose, dry mouth, dry eyes, and excess ear wax.**
- **⅄** **Constipation, diarrhea, hemorrhoids, and gas.**

Make it a habit to compliment your self assessment skills and learn to hone in on your perception skills with regular practice and keen assessment. Record the negative and positive feelings you observe, like how does this or that compare with what you observed the day before. Pay attention to what you may have eaten and of how certain foods made you feel. Take the time to read the subsequent signals and symptoms that may arise at certain times of the day, see what new symptoms you've noticed compared to the old ones. See what parts of the body are affected that weren't before?

Habits play a crucial part in life and human development. The personality of a person is also determined by his or her's habits. There is also no force in the human body that is stronger than one's will power. Therefore you must cultivate the habits of listening to your body and mind by waking up regularly, exercising the body regularly, have healthy eating habits, and to take heed of the valuable information that comes to us through our bodily sensations and emotions. Simply, we just need to learn to pay attention to what is happening in our bodies.

For those of you that have children, make sure their eating healthy to strengthen their immune system. Nutritional deficiencies are very common in children, help protect your child from oncoming illnesses that may occur from improper eating habits. A national study of more than 3,000 US children showed that low vitamin D levels are associated with an increased likely hood that children will develop allergies, according to a paper published Feb 17 by the Journal of Allergy and Clinical Immunology.

This interesting study showed how for example, children who had vitamin D deficiencies, were 2.4 times as likely to have a peanut allergy than were children with sufficient vitamin D levels.
Deficiencies of a nutritional order can cause allergies to specific foods and a hypersensitivity to your immune system. Some of these nutritional deficiencies can be o a inherited disorder some where along the gene pool from your mother or your father's side that's been past down through generations which has never been corrected or found. Also, by supplying the missing nutrient you can correct the specific allergy pertaining to cause of the allergy. In the next chapter, you will find it to be of interest in how you can decode allergies and the specific allergen.

Decoding Your Body's Allergic Symptoms

Allergies are among the most common chronic conditions worldwide that afflict millions of people. An allergy is a hypersensitivity disorder of the immune system. This reaction occurs when a person's immune system reacts to a normally harmless substance in the environment, chemicals, or the types of food we eat. The substance that causes this reaction is called an allergen. This reaction usually results in an inflammatory response which can range from uncomfortable to being dangerous.

There are mild allergies like hay fever that are very common in the human population and cause general symptoms such as red eyes, swollen eyes, itchy eyes, runny nose, eczema, hives, or even an asthma attack. In some people, allergies can play a major role in conditions such as asthma, and severe allergies to environmental or dietary allergens or to medications may result in life-threatening reactions called anaphylaxis shock.

Food allergies, and reactions to the venom of stings from bees, wasps, and insects are often associated with these severe reactions. The typical treatments for allergies include avoiding certain known allergens, use of medications such as anti-histamines that prevent allergic reactions, steroids that modify the immune system in general, and medications such as decongestants that reduce the symptoms. Also there are many in the medical profession that believe allergies to be incurable, in which I tend to disagree. As a aturophathic Practitioner, I believe that every allergy has a nutritional antidote.

utritional research pioneer, Dr. Donald J. Lepore, director of the Life Extension
search Center in Jersey City, N.J. Has conducted successful research using
iokinesiology, herbs, amino acids, vitamins, minerals, and homeopathy having a
putation in succeeding when all else failed. Dr. Lepore believes that every allergy has a
utritional antidote, and uses the term "Metabolic Antagonist" instead of allergy. He
tilizes a technique that he has developed called the "Lepore" technique, which is
asically a fined "muscle response test" technique to accomplish pin pointing the
netabolic antagonist, measure the needed nutrient (nutritional antidote) which could be a
itamin, mineral, herb, cell salt or amino acid remedy to neutralize the metabolic
ntagonist.

le measures the needed support nutrients which are catalysts to assist in the absorption
f the antidote. To learn more about this interesting procedure, you can learn more about
nis in his book called _"The Ultimate Healing System:The Illustrated Guide To Muscle
esting & Nutrition."_

he "Lepore Technique" has proven very successful with many of his clients. Recent
search has been experimenting with this technique and proved to be successful with
nding a nutritional antidote to the many allergies listed. For example, many of the
ommon food allergies that people often experience are caused by the body's inability to
bsorb nutrients because the source of these nutrients is hostile to the body. This hostility
 referred to "Metabolic Antagonism", which is just another way of saying allergy.

hrough 10 years of Dr. Lepore's practice and research, he has found that allergies can be
ured. Unlike what the medical establishment deems that there is no cure for allergies.
hrough research and practice, Dr. Lepore has discovered that each substance that is a
Metabolic Antagonist" or (allergic substance) is caused by or attributed to a certain
utrient, or a combination of nutrient deficiency. Further more, it was found that specific
itamins, minerals, and amino acid combinations are necessary for the complete
bsorption of particular foods.

 typical example allergy to yeast and the nutrient needed to absorb yeast is the mineral
inc. Other vitamins that may also be lacking and could cause ayeast allergy, would be
ie vitamins B1 and B6. And herbs, which can also be used to correct a yeast allergy are
au D' Arco, Red Clover(rich in zinc) and Comfrey. The amino acid that is necessary to
lleviate yeast is Lysine, which is also found in the herb Comfrey.

upplement manufactures also use rice as a base for the manufacturing of multi-vitamins
nd B vitamins, and many of these supplement manufactures do not realize that people
an be allergic to rice. The antidote to a rice allergy is the mineral Manganese, the amino
cids Arginine, proline, and the vitamins B6 (pyrdoxine) and B12 (cyanocobalamine).
nother common allergy is "Wheat." Vitamins such as vitamin E are often made from
vheat germ and are not properly absorb by the person with the wheat allergy. Antidotes
 wheat allergy is Magnesium, Histidine, and vitamin F (linoleic acid) which also
ontains vitamin E. It should be also noted that those with feather and wool allergies will
lso respond to the wheat antidotes – magnesium, histidine, sodium, and vitamin F.

The next common allergy is the Fat Allergy" and is usually caused by the lack of the mineral sulfur. An over consumption of fatty foods can deplete the body of sulfur and will create a fat allergy. The two significant factors that can contribute to a fat allergy is from people who smoke and live in a polluted environment. Sulfur is an important mineral as it helps the body purify the blood from smoking, and many other impurities that we may take in by being exposed to environmental pollutants. The symptoms of a sulfur deficiency is lots of phlem in the throat, congestion in the lungs and a heaviness in the chest near the thymus gland. Your tonsils may also be inflamed and are basically the sulfur sack of the body.

The antidote to a fat allergy are the amino acids methionine, Cysteine, Taurine, and Glutathione are all very good sources of sulfur. The herbs that are good sources of sulfur are Sarsaparilla, Fenugreek, dandelion, Burdock and Fennel seeds. The homeopathic Sulfur 1-x potency cell salt is also helpful in correcting a fat allergy condition and can sometimes bring on quick relief. It was also found that exposure to the sun can help clear up a fat allergy as well. Other suggested sources include the consumption of certain food like bananas, eggs, garlic, onions, and the amino acid Threonine.

Another common allergy that is related to the wheat allergy, is corn, occurring when there is a lack of Potassuim. The corn allergy can occur when there is a lack of the vitamin F, magnesium, and histidine. Those that are allergic to corn should be aware of vitamin pills that are coated with a "zien" coating which is actually a corn based coating.

A lack of iron can provoke an allergy to oatmeal and sesame. Babies that are fed oatmeal sometimes get colic from it which is a allergic response due to the lack of iron in their blood. One of the best natural sources of iron is the herb Yellow Dock, and can also be corrected by vitamins B12, amino acid citrilline, and folic acid.

The next common allergy is the "Milk" allergy. This can be corrected by the mineral Potassium. Milk and milk by-products can all be allergic if there is a deficiency of Potassium. The amino acid Aspartic acid and the vitamin D can also help correct milk intolerance. Citrus allergies are also common and can be corrected with vitamin B5 (pantothenic acid). Vitamin B5 can become deficient very easily due to unrelenting stress levels which can deplete your B5 levels quite fast which often results in the citrus allergy. Therefore, stress or trauma can actually create a citrus allergy. The mineral antidote for a citrus allergy is Calcium and the amino acid is Serine. One of the best natural sources of B5 is Royal Jelly.

An allergies to peppers is caused by a deficiency of niacin vitamin B3 and the mineral Phosphorus, and the amino acid Glutamine. It was also found that when a persons sodium and potassium levels have been depleted, they normally become allergic to every thing. Good natural sources of potassium are bee pollen, alfalfa which also contains both the sodium and potassium. It should also be noted that if a person becomes potassium depleted, milk, cheese and all foods that contain sodium would become allergic. Of all the vitamins and minerals, potassium and sodium tend to be the most unstable since they are burned up so quickly. Stress too can also cause a potassium and sodium loss from the body because stress affects the adrenal glands which create a need for these two minerals.

Allergies are just another way of our body's warning signs that something is wrong and ery allergen has its antidote, just like every nutritional deficiency has its symptoms. llergies are nothing more than our body informing us that what we are consuming lacks certain nutritional compound to help in its metabolic conversion to benefit our ltritional need. Deficiencies are becoming more and more widespread in this country, d it will benefit us if we can understand and interpret the various signs and symptoms the prevention of a long term health problem that may manifest. I also find it amazing w deficiencies in two important minerals like sodium and potassium can create so any allergies to the different amount of foods we eat on a daily basis.

his just goes to show how important minerals our to our health and well being. Science also starting to realize how certain cancers are related to the vital minerals our body :eds to sustain life. You must also realize and take note that from the minerals our body nsumes helps in the manufacturing of vitamins and the metabolism of amino acids. ciety in today's world must realize how our food chain is being devoid of nutrients om the foods we grow, weather has played a major part in the erosion of top soil ashing away the fertile soil and lea ving most of the ground barren with empty rtilization that is needed in the growth of vegetables, and the grass that our animal eat well.

many of the products that we buy in the grocery store has been fortified or enhanced ith certain vitamins and minerals. Our meats have also been contaminated with steroids, r crops are sprayed with pesticides and chemicals, thus weakening and contaminating r nutritional means of health. Organic goods now cost more than regular foods, where years ago it was a common practice of all natural foods.

he bottom line is to try and eat as healthy as you can and know when your body is ying to tell you a warning sign that it may be lacking certain nutrients that it may need function on an optimal level. Allergies are just another way our body's are trying to tell something, you can see by now how being deficient in certain nutrients can affect the etabolism of the foods being consumed. Every symptom, sign, or signal that are body's ve off, there's a reason and a remedy at hand.

e smart and be safe, learn how to read these messages and prevent illness from anifesting. Study the recommended books on muscle response testing, and the signs d symptoms when your body tries to talk to you. Pay attention to the foods that you nsume daily and make notes on how it makes you feel. These easy little techniques can along way in preventing yourself from visiting an UN-necessary trip to the nergency room.

y utilizing the muscle response testing protocol, you can assess many of the common lergens that can be causing your specific allergy. You would be surprised how accurate e results can be, and remember, prevention is the ultimate cure in disease manifestion. or those of you that are interested in learning more of Dr. Lepore's technique, I highly commend that you read his book - *"The Ultimate Healing System:The Illustrated Guide o Muscle Testing & Nutrition."* and for information on muscle response testing called - Healing Energies" by Dr. Stephen Paul Shepard.

Decoding Food Allergies and Their Specific Neutralizing Nutrient

<u>Food Allergy</u> > <u>Vitamins</u> > <u>Minerals</u> > <u>Amino Acids</u> > <u>Herb's</u>

<u>Yeast</u> > Vitamin B1 (thiamine) > Zinc > Lysine > Red Clover & Comfrey
- Barley > (same for all below)
- Millet
- Potatoes
- Prunes
- Raisins
- Rye
- Walnuts

<u>Rice</u> > B6, B12 > Manganese > Arginine, Proline > Yucca Plant, Beet powder.
- Curry (same for all below)
- Cinnamon
- Blueberries
- Grapes
- Straw berries
- Watermelon
- Wine
- Pumpkin

<u>Wheat</u> > Essential Fatty Acids (vit-F) Omega 3's >Magnesium > Histidine >Black Walnut
- Feathers
  Kelp
- Wool
  Spirulina
- Dust
- Detergents
- Dander (cats & dogs)

<u>Corn</u> > Essential Fatty Acids> Magnesium, Potassium>Histidine> Black Walnut, Kelp and Bee Pollen

<u>Meat Fats</u> > Biotin>Carnitine>Sulfur>Methionine, Cysteine, Taurine, Glutathione and

<u>Milk Fats Threonine</u> > Sarsaparilla,Eyebright, Dandelion, Burdock, Fennel Seeds.

<u>Vegetables</u>

<u>Cosmetics</u>

<u>Oatmeal</u> > Folic Acid, B12 > Iron > Citrulline > Yellow Dock

<u>Sesame</u>

<u>Milk & Cheese</u> > Vitamin D >Potassium>Aspartic Acid> Asparagine>Bee pollen,Alfalfa and Hawthorne Berries.

itrus >Vitamin B5 > Calcium> Serine > Royal Jelly

eppers > Vitamin B3 > Phosphorus > L-Glutamine > Royal Jelly
eaches
ears
lums
ectarines

ote: Sometimes food intolerance's or allergies can also be due to missing enzymes the digestive system that prevents a person from fully digesting the food. Also, od posioning can have toxins or bacteria that make you sick, to which just because me particular food makes you sick doesn't mean you're allergic to it, although it ould be checked out by a physician to eliminate the particular cause.

ther possible causes are food additives like MSG (monosodium-glutamate) and lfites often cause bad reactions in some people which in most cases is a chemical action to the additive, not the food itself.

often wondered many years ago, why am I so lucky with any unknown allergies to any ods or any environmental and chemical allergic reactions, when my wife and best iend have some of the specific common allergies that every one else may have. I guess may be genetics and good wholesome nutrition during my childhood years, plus living n a farm and eating fresh organic foods and livestock had a lot to do with it.

his has to explain why some people are allergic and some are not. Honestly we are all e same flesh and blood, human beings from different mothers and fathers. This goes ack to biochemical individuality, where we are all different nutritionally. For every ause, there's an action, and for every allergy, there's an antidote.

When you're allergic to some specific food or chemical, the body's immune system ecognizes the allergen and reacts to it by producing antibodies to counter act it. lentifying it as a harmful substance or an invader to the body. This reaction releases uge stores of "Histamine" which causes symptoms ranging from a mild case of hives to potentially life threatening system shutdown. Obviously, if there is a nutritional void or n enzyme that's required in the metabolism of the specific food eaten, there is going to e an allergic response. Your body will react by either a skin rash, hives,watery swollen yes, headaches, hypersensitivity, a rise in blood pressure, and anaphylaxis shock.

quick way of determining if your allergic to a specific food is to check your pulse rate, ormally it will rise and beat faster. The other type of allergy test are skin tests – with a kin test, the skin is scratched or pricked with a tiny bit of liquid extract of an allergen uch as pollen or food). If the area of the skin swells up and becomes red (like a osquito bite), the test is said to be positive, meaning that your allergic to that substance. kin testing allows you to see within 15 minutes if your allergic to the substances tested. lood tests are also used by doctors, but they take a few days to get the results back.

Warning Sign's of Metal Toxicity

There is one particular allergen that goes by undetected in so many people and can cause many health problems from A to Z, which is a wonder why our government allows its use? And that is "Amalgam Fillings" used once by so many dentists in this country. I once had a client come and see me for her bad allergies that she was having. She explained to me that her allergy was due to her two Siamese cats that she was very fond of. What was interesting was, that prior to owning the cats she was never allergic to them before and that was after several years of owning the two cats.

She also explained that she had seen several allergy specialists in Manhattan, NYC. And they had prescribed several scripts and anti-allergy shots to help support her allergy problems, which didn't seem to help her. They also told her to her disappointment to get rid of her two Siamese cats that she loved and cared for. Well, I was her last hope! After analyzing her health questionnaire, I recommended that she take a *"hair tissue mineral analysis test"* to help determine any nutritional deficiencies that she may have had and to check for any accumulations of toxic metals in her blood stream that may be causing her immune system to reject the specific allergens she was having.

Within two weeks her analysis test came back and it was discovered that she had high levels of mercury poisoning that was causing her to become allergic to her two cats. And this was due to her amalgam fillings that she had from years ago. Problem solved, once she returned back to her dentist and removed the fillings, she was no longer allergic to her cats and was very happy and ecstatic to be able to hold her animals once again!

The point here is why is our government allowing toxic metals to be used in dentistry that can harm us? Mercury is the most toxic non-radioactive metal on earth! It has been well known that mercury is dangerous. Its dangerous to touch and even more so to ingest. But never the less, the American dental Association (ADA) has convinced dentists, the US government, and the American people that once mercury is combined with other substances in an amalgam filling, it becomes perfectly safe.

This is incredibly ironic, considering that this very same amalgam mixture (including amalgam fillings removed from peoples mouths) must be handled, transported and disposed of as a "toxic substance". How can they explain their reasoning that amalgam suddenly becomes perfectly safe once placed in the volatile environment of the human mouth, and then dangerous again when removed? Well the answer is the same as any answer surrounded by corruption and shrouded by misinformation, money and according to Hal Huggins, one of the men leading the fight to remove mercury from dental fillings in the United States. The ADA makes about $50 million per year from royalties associated with the manufacturing of amalgam fillings.

Mercury is related to numerous health issues that defies normal health care. Evidence and research – both old and new shows that mercury causes or plays a significant role in so many health issues too numerous for me to list! Do yourself a favor and just look up the health problems that mercury fillings can cause, you would be very surprised and astonished that our government would allow such a thing.

Next time when your having difficulties in trying to determine your health related problem that you, nor your doctor can come to the conclusion of, (just like my client with allergies to her cats) to check and see if you have any mercury amalgam fillings that were one years ago and forgotten about. It can affect or mask any of the diseases currently spread throughout the US. It is amazing how so many diseases – both physical and mental may originate just from amalgam fillings. And how many more people throughout this country walk around every day with chronic ailments that their body is suffering from unknowingly with test after test with no resolvement what so ever!

This is no different than my client developing allergies she never had before, seeing specialist after specialist that never bothered to check for certain toxic substances in the body. Just about every other American in this country will show some kind of minor or major toxicity in their bloodstream. Our food chain is loaded with toxic metals, that can be found in everything from tooth paste, cosmetics, foods in cans and boxes and many more related items that we consume and use on a daily basis. Mercury exposure can also come other sources like – shellfish, tuna, water proof mascara, hair dyes, hemorrhoid medicines, gardening chemicals, and many more. It makes one wonder if the United States government is literally try to poison us for the mere sake of profit!

The bottom line is, If you do suspect that you may have mercury poisoning, you can find a doctor that is skilled in this area, or just go to your dentist and have your fillings replaced.

For more information on mercury poisoning see the book "*Amalgam Illness*" that provides incredible detail and information on this subject.

Well enough said, I hope you get the message? And this could make for another book on The Conspiracy Factor: Is Our Government Trying To Poison Us?" Remember, when no known cause for disease or illness can be found, it is important to look for a hidden body of burden to toxic metals. Examples of these metals include mercury, lead, aluminum, arsenic, and cadium(cigarrtte smoke).

Some of these metals can also get into your body through drinking polluted water, dental fillings breathing contaminated air or eating foods that may be exposed to dangerous metals. Mercury, aluminum, and arsenic are some of the three toxic metals normally found in some foods in trace amounts that can build up over time and can impair brain function.

Signs and Symptoms of Metal Poisoning

Heavy metal poisoning and chemical toxicity can lead to the accumulation of toxins in our tissues and organs causing nutritional deficiencies, hormonal imbalances , and the breakdown of the immune system, the central nervous system, and the organs of the body. This breakdown of bodily organs and systems will encourage numerous diseases and disorders to take hold in the body.

It is important to know some of the early warning signs and symptoms of these toxins so that you can take action and reverse it. The one most important fact that people take for granted in this modern toxic world is cleaning the inside of our bodies, our colon (the sewer system of the body), our liver, and other organs require regular cleaning just like a car requires an oil change once and awhile. Every day we shower, brush our teeth, wash our hair on a regular basis, but how many people remember to do the same on the inside?

Some of you may ask, well how do we know when its time to clean our inside to free our body of accumulated toxins, parasites and other waste materials? You should basically do a body detox every three months or so to make sure your internals are functioning optimally. And if our body could talk, the signs and many symptoms it warn you of would be as follows:

- Bad breath & foul-smelling stools
- Brain fog
- Coated tongue
- Extreme fatigue Food allergies
- Frequent colds
- Insomnia
- Loss of memory
- Metallic taste in mouth
- Muscle twitching
- Muscle & joint pain
- Night sweats
- Parasites
- Powerful food cravings
- Recurring headaches
- Skin problems, rashes
- Sore or receding gums
- Sensitivity to smells
- Irritability, mood swings
- and many more others!

The two major symptoms of chemical & heavy metal toxicity are the breakdown of the immune system and diseases of the organs and central nervous system. The first thing often recommended for anyone who is experiencing symptoms of metal poisoning is to have a **"hair mineral analysis test"** done. A hair analysis can determine which toxic heavy metals your body has been excreting and can give you an excellent baseline before you embark on any type of heavy metal cleansing or detoxification program. Regular blood tests and urine tests are not accurate in diagnosing heavy metal toxicity, as they only tend to show what is happening in the body at that brief moment in time, and do not give you the long term picture.

The hair analysis will also tell you which essential minerals your body is needing more of and which mineral ratios are imbalanced due to heavy metals, and also provides valuable insight into your metabolism and what dietary changes might be helpful. This test can provide you with much needed information about mineral deficiencies and imbalances in your body, especially if you are suffering from symptoms of heavy metal poisoning. It's highly recommended!

The following is a list of the most common disorders found by independent research studies to be directly linked to toxic metals and chemicals.

Disorders Linked to Heavy Metal Poisoning and Chemical Toxicity

- ADD - Schizophrenia
- Autism
- Alzheimer's Disease-Parkinson's Disease
- Asthma
- Cancer
- Arthritis
- Heart Disease
- Gulf War Syndrome
- Epilepsy
- Auto-Immune Disorders – Chronic Fatigue-Fibromyalgia-
- Multiple Sclerosis-ALS
- Insomnia
- Hypertension
- Liver Disease
- Infertility
- Thyroid Disorders

Natural Methods for Detoxifying Metal Toxins & Chemicals

The following list of products are a safe alternative to traditional chelators used in chelation therapy for removing heavy metals and chemical pollutants. These chelating agents create a chemical bond with these metals to make them less active and combine in the blood stream to successfully excrete them through your **kidneys and liver**.

Milk Thistle – Helps your liver detoxify and in the process, eliminates heavy metals. Milk thistle also helps heal and cleanse the liver of impurities.

Chlorella – Used in the orient for heavy metal detoxification and helps to purify the bloodstream.

Glutathione – An important amino acid that is considered to be the body's master anti-oxidant and detoxifying agent. A major player in detoxifying the body of many pollutants, including toxic metals and chemicals. Just by having a Glutathione deficiency will impair the body's ability to get rid of toxins whether they are of environmental or the by-product of cellular metabolism.

Vitamin B6 – is advised if you have under gone dental procedures or have dental fillings. It prevents the contamination of heavy metals in the body.

Epsom Salt Bath – An excellent way to help your body leach out the toxins from the body. Rich in the mineral Magnesium Sulphate, when it is absorbed through the skin, such as in a bath, it draws out toxins, sedates the nervous system, reduces swelling, relaxes muscles, is a natural emollient, exfoliator, and much more!

Alpha Lipoic Acid- a potent anti-oxidant that is both water and fat soluble and passes through the blood brain and has been also shown to chelate metals like mercury that can attach to fatty cells and brain neurons. It also deceases metals from the liver as well.

Vitamin C & E – Together these two supplements enhance each other's effectiveness as a detoxifying agent. The combination of the two vitamins inhibits free radical damage and activity that increases while carrying a heavy metal burden, the presence of one prolongs the presence of the other.

The quality of your health depends upon many pieces that not only includes the health of your bodily systems, but also includes a healthy diet, exercise, and spirituality. Make some key adjustments by including foods rich in **anti-oxidants like vitamins A, C, E, beta carotene**, that defend you against heavy metal build up. Include more citrus fruits like oranges, tangerines, grapefruits, lemons and eat foods that can increase your **Glutathione (GSH)** levels such as asparagus, broccoli, and spinach. Supplements like pure **100% whey protein** rich in amino acids can help raise your glutathione levels as well.

Eating lots of **fiber** is another effective way of preventing heavy metals from being absorbed, add ground flax seeds to your meals can help also by promoting digestive regularity. Foods rich in **omega 3's such as flax seed oil, fish oils, wild salmon, avocados, and sprouted walnuts**. Try an add cilantro to your diet, as anecdotal evidence suggests that cilantro may help mobilize mercury and other toxic metals, pulling them out of the brain to more superficial structures where they can be more easily grabbed and excreted by chelating agents. And drink purified water throughout the day by keeping the body well hydrated to help flush out impurities from the kidney's. Learn to stay away from drinking tap water to reduce your exposure to many metals found in tap water.

Eliminate sugar and sugar by products – candy, cookies, cakes, juices, soda's,etc., Limit your use of alcohol as it impairs your immune and detoxification systems. Stay away from saturated fats and many of the processed foods. Learn also to cook with aluminum free pots and pans, choose stainless steel instead. Avoid drinking from aluminum cans, and avoid the use of aluminum foil in food preservation or cooking. By learning to take the necessary precautions about heavy metal build up in the body, will help you and your family less likely to be exposed to the toxicity of metal build up that can cause a host of ill health diseases.

General Detoxification & Body Cleansing

Toxic exposure has recently become a great concern among society today and I will go on and say that the toxicity that threatens our health from the foods we eat, cosmetics we use, to the water we drink, and the air we breathe creates the perfect scenario for cancers, allergies, and disease manifestations. The average American now eats 9 pounds of chemicals annually, consumes 150 lbs of sugar a year, and the average autopsy reports 5 pounds of undigested meat in the intestines as well.

The list of these foreign materials in our food includes a host of - *additives, preservatives, dyes, bleaches, emulsifiers, acidifiers, alkalizers, fortifiers, sweeteners, hydrolizers, drying agents,* and list goes on and on! And of the 60,000 chemicals in general use today, fewer than 2% have been tested for safety. Every day we ingest more of these food chemicals that can increase the incidence of allergies and degenerative diseases like; cancers, diabetes, multiple sclerosis, heart disease, and diseases of the liver

nd kidney. In 1900's, the death rate from cancer was one person out of every 30. Now it
ills one person out of five, and in heart disease, it killed one person out of every seven,
ow it includes one out of every two persons. There's a connection to be made between
ncreased toxicity and increases in diseases, the answer is fairly obvious.

oxicity occurs on two basic levels – internally and externally. Internally our body
ormally produces toxins from every day functions and cellular activity, which are called
ee radicals (biochemical toxins). If these toxins are not counteracted or eliminated, they
an irritate and inflame our cells and bodily tissues. Even our thoughts and emotions, and
specially stress can increase biochemical toxicity.

lmost everyone needs to detox and cleanse their body from time to time. Detoxification
nd cleansing can contribute to the healing of many acute and chronic illnesses. Give
our body a clean fresh start by applying a cleansing program to feel more alive and
ore aware. In doing so you will begin to feel a new sense of vitality, improved
emory, clearer skin, enhanced senses, rest your organs, improve weight loss, be more
roductive, creative, motivated, and most importantly prevent disease!

The Non-Toxic Diet

he non toxic diet provides for you a preventive way of medicine to follow to try and
void toxicity. This allows you to learn ways to create and support a healthy lifestyle.
he first step is to employ a whole body cleanse – internally and externally. And your
on toxic diet should be to – *eat organic foods whenever possible, drink filtered water,
otate the common allergen foods like milk products, wheat, and yeast by products* (see
hapter on antidotes to allergies)*, practice food combining; Include fruits, veg's,
hole grains, legumes, nuts, seeds, fresh fish(no shell-fish), and organic poultry.*

*ook in iron, stainless steel pots & pans, glass, or porcelain cookware. Avoid or
inimize red meats, cured meats, organ meats, refined foods, canned & boxed foods,
ugar, regular table salt(sea salt is good), saturated fats, excess coffee, alcohol and
icotine.*

olon cleansing is one of the most important steps in detoxification. Helpful products
nclude the herbal laxatives, fiber and colon detox supplements such as psyllium seed
usks alone or mixed with aloe vera powder and acidophilus culture. Enemas using
ater, herbs, or diluted black coffee which stimulates liver cleansing, may also be used.
r you can employ a series of colonic water irrigation done by a trained professional,
hich can be a focal point of a body detoxification program along with a cleansing diet
nd fiber supplements.

Vhat ever method you use it is important to keep the bowels moving is the key to feeling
vell during the detox program. Regular exercise is also very important as it stimulates
weating and encourages elimination through the skin and strengthens your muscles and
nternal organs. Regular aerobic exercise is another one of the keys in maintaining a
ontoxic body. **Epsom salt** baths are also commonly used along with skin brushing while
athing.

axative and colon cleansing herbs that are good to use are – **cascara sagrada,**

dandelion, buckthorn, senna leaf, yellow dock, and licorice.

Liver cleansers – **Milk thistle, amino acid taurine, dandelion and globe artichoke. Healthy vegetables for liver health – carrots, pumpkins, bell peppers, and beets.**

Great Liver Tonic – **"Livatone"**, contains important herbs and amino acids plus **B vitamins** and lipotropic co-factors essential for healthy liver function and detoxification

Kidney Cleansers – herbs that help to flush out impurities and detox the kidneys are – **juniper berries, parsley, uva ursi, cranberry extract, dandelion, watermelon seeds, celery and asparagus.**

Detoxification – What To Expect

In the process of cleansing and rebuilding, some people may experience some discomfort, such as headaches, nausea, indigestion, diarrhea, or fatigue. Usually these symptoms pass in 3 to 5 days or so and happen because of toxins that are temporarily being dumped faster than the body can eliminate them. Its a lot like house cleaning, when you take up a broom and start to suddenly stir up a dust storm. Drinking more pure water usually helps this adjustment period to pass more quickly.

A quick important word about water – our life, our planet and over 70% of the earth's surface is covered in water. Water is the basis of all life, your muscles that move your body is 75% water; your blood that transports nutrients is 82% water, your lungs that provide oxygen are 90% water; your brain that is the control center of your body is 76% water; and even your bones are 25% water. It provides the medium in which all biochemical reactions take place in the body. Water is needed to eliminate wastes through the kidneys, colon and the skin. Most people do not generally consume enough pure water to properly hydrate the body. Make it a healthy habit and consume two liters of pure water daily, if you truly are committed to a healthy lifestyle. It is a free investment for your long-term health!

Note: Investing in a home reverse osmosis unit can ensure the purity of most drinking water.

For those interested in a more thorough body cleanse, I recommend "The Liver Cleansing Diet" by Dr. Sandra Cabot.

Detoxification isn't necessarily fun but it is necessary. Listen to the warning signs your body is sending you! Be grateful that your body in its divine wisdom is giving you that headache, cold, body ache, or pain. Don't try to suppress them, but instead learn to what the warning signs mean.

Warning Signs That Indicate Medical Emergency

The most 'urgent" or red-light signals and symptoms that could spell a trip to the emergency room often manifest quite readily at times and should be addressed immediately to prevent a serious oncoming health condition or a life-threatening one.

ccording to Doctor's Neil Shulman,MD, Jack Birge,MD, and Joon Ahn,MD, the three eorgia based doctors that are the authors of the book *"Your Body's Red Light Warning ignals"* - They state that certain medical symptoms and signals are warning you of otential health problems that are considered "Red-Light" signals that requires nmediate care, as soon as possible! Such as :

"Urgent" Warning Signs Related To The Brain

Headaches – A sudden, agonizing and pounding headache – the worst of your life, ould mean <u>bleeding in the brain.</u>(if you have these symptoms call 911).

Strokes – Strokes happen when blood flow to the brain stops or is suddenly npaired and within minutes brain cells begin to die. There are also two kinds of trokes, the more common is "Ischemic Stroke" - caused by a blood clot that blocks r plugs a blood vessel in the brain. The other kind of stroke is called "Hemorrhagic troke", is caused by a blood vessels that breaks and bleeds into the brain. *ymptoms are - sudden loss of feeling in the arms or legs, tingling, numbness, isorientation, slurred speech, your face appears droopy, trouble blinking, double ision, dizziness, and weakness, especially on one side of the body. (if you have these ymptoms call 911)*

Major symptoms are> sudden onset of slurred speech> droopy face> trouble linking>can't move a limb or arms>feeling weak & numbness> and last a severe eadache!

Brain Aneurysm – Sometimes called 'berry aneurysm" because often are the size of small berry. A brain aneurysm is an "abnormal bulge or ballooning" in the wall of n artery in the brain. Most brain aneurysms produce no symptoms until they ecome quite large, and begin to leak blood or rupture. <u>A brain aneurysm will roduce signs when it presses on the nerves of the brain, which can cause the ollowing</u> *symptoms – A droopy eye lid, double vision, pain above or behind the eye, a ilated pupil, numbness or weakness on one side of the face or body.(if so call 911)*

Urgent Warning Signs Of The Body

Heart Attacks – The early warning sign of a heart attack – *are chest pain or iscomfort with pain in the arm, jaw, or neck; breaking out in a cold sweat, extreme veakness, nausea, vomiting, feeling faint, or being short of breath. (if so call 911 mmediately).*

Pulmonary Embolisms – A sudden blockage in a lung artery, usually caused by a lood clot in the leg called deep vein thrombosis that breaks loose and travels hrough the blood stream to the lungs. This is a serious condition that can cause – ermanent damage to the affected lung, lower oxygen levels in your blood, and lamage other vital organs in your body from not getting enough oxygen.

Note: half of the people who have pulmonary embolism have no symptoms. If you lo have *symptoms they can include – shortness of breath, chest pain or coughing up lood, and swelling, pain, tenderness and redness of the leg affected from the blood*

clot. If the blood clot is large, or if there are many clots, pulmonary embolism can
cause death! (Seek immediate care, call 911)

Blood Clots - _Symptom are tenderness and pain in the back of your lower legs,_
swollen calf muscles and tender to the touch, chest pain, shortness of breath, or
coughing up blood. These symptoms can be the result of a potentially dangerous
blood clot in your leg, especially if they come after you've been sitting or lying down
for prolonged periods of time, such as on an airplane or during a long car trip. This
can cause blood to pool in your legs when your sitting or lying down for long
periods of time, as opposed to standing and walking. If you get a sudden chest pain
and shortness of breath, a piece of the blood clot may have traveled through the
blood stream to your lungs. Blood clots can be life threatening, so seek emergency
care! And call 911.

Blood in Urine – Can always be a serious condition any time you see blood in your
urine, even if there is no pain present, you should call your doctor promptly. Blood
in your urine can be caused by kidney stones, bladder infections, or a prostate
infection. And possibly worst, cancer of the kidney, ureter, bladder, or prostate.
Don't dismiss this important sign , and take a wait and see approach as most people
often do, thinking this is a one time occurrence and may not cause any pain. Blood
in the urine may be the only clue for an early diagnosis and cure!

Asthma Attacks – This happens when asthma attacks are worse and don't subside.
Asthma attacks are marked by wheezing and difficulty in breathing. When attacks
happen and don't improve, seek immediate medical attention and call 911. Left
untreated, it could result in severe chest muscle fatigue and death. Asthma makes
breathing difficult, and as a result their blood oxygen levels drops while blood levels
of carbon dioxide rises having a sedating affect on the brain causing them to feel
even drowsier.

Note: A person with asthma who seems to be relaxing more, and seems not to be
struggling for breath anymore – even though they've been at it for 6 or 8 hours may
actually be worse. This could be a sign of respiratory fatigue, according to doctors
Jack Birge, MD, and Neil Schulman, MD and authors of the book "Your Body's
Red Light Warning Signals".

Anaphylactic Shock - Is a widespread and very serious allergic reaction that can
become fatal! Symptoms include - labored breathing, dizziness, swelling of the
tongue and breathing tubes, blueness of skin, loss of consciousness, low blood
pressure, heart failure and death. Anaphylactic shock requires immediate
emergency treatment including administration of anti-venom in the case of bee or
wasp stings, or epinephrine depending on the type of allergen. Either case call 911
immediately.

Sleep Apnea – Literally means, "without breath during sleep." Clinically, it means
that patients are actually _stopping their breathing pattern periodically throughout the_
night while sleeping. Symptoms can be – _excessive daytime sleepiness, frequent_
episodes of obstructed breathing (made aware of, by the bed partner).

hese episodes are normally brief, and happen before the body protectively wakes p enough to restart the breathing pattern again. <u>Sleep apnea could be a potentially fe threatening condition that requires immediate medical attention.</u> *The risks of ndiagnosed obstructive sleep apnea include – heart attacks, strokes, irregular heart eat, high blood pressure and heart disease. In addition, sleep apnea causes daytime eepiness that can result in accidents.*

n official diagnosis of sleep apnea may require seeing a sleep specialist and a ome-based sleep-test using portable monitors or an over night stay at the hospital. nyone can have sleep apnea – young, old, male or female, and even children can uffer. However, certain risk factors have been associated with obstructive and entral sleep apnea. <u>You can also have a higher risk for obstructive sleep apnea if ou are</u> - – related to someone that has sleep apnea, over the age of 65, Black, Iispanic, or a Pacific Islander, a smoker, male, and over weight.

ppendicitis Attack – *<u>Abdominal pain and tenderness that may first appear around ie belly button and then move toward the lower right area of the abdomen are the iain symptoms.</u> Other common signs and symptoms include – pain that gets worse hen moving, taking deep breaths, coughing and sneezing; low fever that begins after ther symptoms, abdominal swelling, nausea, vomiting, inability to pass gas, feeling ke a bowel movement will relieve the discomfort, and loss of appetite. <u>If you xperience these possible signs call 911 and seek medical emergency.</u>* ppendicitis normally occurs when bacteria invade and infect the wall of the ppendix.

iabetic Shock – *Symptoms include a sweet, chemical odor on the patient's breath that : similar to that of acetone or alcohol (acetone breath), fatigue, light headedness or iinting, and often reddening of the skin. <u>Resulting from extremely low blood sugar ssociated with diabetes.</u>* Immediate treatment of glucose in a prescription sub-ngual form, or even hard candy or orange juice if nothing else is available. Patients ı a state of diabetic shock should also be evaluated medically immediately after mergency treatment. If left untreated, this condition will lead to coma and even eath. <u>ymptoms of low blood sugar typically appear when the sugar levels falls below 0mg/dl and include – weakness, shakiness, sweating, headaches, nervousness, and unger.</u> Low blood sugar levels can also occur when the patient use's too much ısulin, exercises for too long, or has not eaten enough food.

Jrgent warning signs are are an ordeal that hopefully we won't have to face someday, but ַ we do, it would be nice to know what these warning signs are. he American College of Emergency Physicians recommends that there are five warning igns or **" Red Flags"** that should not be ignored, which can be of an extreme medical mergency!

1. **Chest Pains** > Any kind of chest pain should be considered a trip to the emergency room. Chest pains can be a sign of a heart attack.

2. **Neurological changes** > Having trouble with your speech all of a sudden and your face feels droopy, your having trouble talking, blinking, and

difficulty moving your arms, you feel weak and numbness could all be a sign of a stroke.

3. **Severe Headache** **that feels like the worst you've had** > Everyone gets headaches or migraines once a month or so, but if it is a headache that's totally different than what your used to, that's an emergency! Go to the E.R. Room right away! Could possible be aneurysm or stroke.

4. **Struggling To Breathe** > Having trouble breathing is not considered normal and should seek emergency medical care immediately! Any form of breathing, either standing, walking, climbing stairs or while you are talking and feel short of breath requires immediate medical care.

5. **Severe Abdominal Pain** > Any pain from the chest on down to the pelvi that is not going away, can be a whole host of medical problems. The sooner you get to the emergency room the better!

Other Vital Medical Emergency Warning Signs

1. **Fainting, sudden dizziness, and weakness.**
2. **Changes in vision.**
3. **Confusion or changes in mental status, unusuall behavior, and difficulty walking.**
4. **Uncontrolled bleeding.**
5. **Severe or persistent vomiting or diarrhea.**
6. **Coughing or vomiting blood.**
7. **Unusual abdominal pain.**
8. **Suicidal or homicidal feelings.**

Note: **knowing what to do in medical emergencies and being prepared can mean th world of a difference in preventive ill health and life threatening situations. You ca learn to recognize and act on emergency warning signs by taking a first aid class and learning CPR at your local hospital, American Red Cross or American Heart Association.**

COMMON CAUSES OF VITAMIN & MINERAL DEFICIENCY GUIDE
"I Told I Was Sick!"

Overview of Vitamins:

Vitamins and minerals were given their name because they are considered essential for optimal health, hence the term *"vital-minerals" equals "vita-mins"*. Vitamins are classified for their biological value and chemical activity, not their structure. They have diverse biochemical functions. Some have hormone-like functions as regulators of mineral metabolism *(e.g.,vitamin D),* or regulators of cell and tissue growth and differentation *(e.g. vitamin A)*. others function as *anti-oxidants (e.g., vitamin E, vitamin C, the mineral selenium and zinc).*

The largest number of vitamins are the *B complex vitamins* which function as precursor or enzyme co-factors, that help enzymes in their work as catalysts in the metabolism. For example, *Biotin is part of an enzymes* involved in making *fatty acids*. Another is *folic acid*, which carries various forms of a carbon group – *methyl, formyl, and methylene in the cell*. All these roles in assisting enzyme-substrate reactions are vitamins best known function, the other vitamin functions are equally important.

extracted from food, vitamins are essential for the growth and development of a multicellular organism. Through genetic blueprint inherited from its parents, a fetus begins to develop, at the moment of conception, from the nutrients it absorbs from the mother. It requires certain vitamins and minerals to be present at certain times. These nutrients facilitate the chemical reactions that produce among other things, skin, bone, muscle and muscle. If there is serious deficiencies in one or more of these nutrients, a child may develop a deficiency disease. Even minor deficiencies may cause permanent damage. Humans can produce some vitamins from the precursors they consume. *Example vitamin A, produced from beta-carotene, and niacin, from the amino acid Tryptophan.*

Once normal growth and development are completed, vitamins and minerals remain essential nutrients for the healthy maintenance of the cells, tissues, and organs that make up a multi-cellular organism. They also enable a multi-cellular life form to efficiently use chemical energy provided by food it eats, and helps process the proteins, carbohydrates, and fats required for respiration.

Vitamins In Humans

Vitamins are also classified as either being **water soluble or fat soluble**. In humans there are *13 vitamins: 4 fat-soluble (A, D, E,and K) and 9 water-soluble (8 B vitamins and vitamin C).* Water soluble vitamins dissolve easily and , in general, are absorbed and excreted from the body, to the degree that urinary output is a strong indicator of vitamin consumption. Because water soluble vitamins are not as readily stored, a more consistent intake is important in maintaining bodily health. Fat soluble vitamins are absorbed through the intestinal tract with the help of lipids (fats). Because they are more likely to accumulate in the body, they are also more likely to lead to hyper-vitaminosis than are the water soluble vitamins.

Importance of Dietary Minerals & Trace Minerals

Overview:
Dietary minerals (also known as mineral nutrients) are the chemical elements required by living organisms, with the four elements being carbon, hydrogen, nitrogen, and oxygen that are present in common organic molecules. Minerals in the order of abundance in the human body include the seven major minerals – *calcium, phosphorus, potassium, sulfur, sodium, chlorine, and magnesium.* Important Trace minerals, necessary for mammalian life, include – *iron, cobalt, copper, zinc, molybdenum, iodine, and selenium.*

All nutrients such as *vitamins, proteins, enzymes, amino acids, carbohydrates, fats, sugars, oils,* etc. require minerals for proper cellular function. All bodily functions depend upon the action and presence of minerals. Acting as catalysts for many biological reactions within the human body, they are necessary for the transmission of messages through the nervous system, digestive system, and the metabolism or utilization of all nutrients in foods. They are most important factors in maintaining all physiological processes, are constituents of the teeth, bones, tissues, blood, muscle, and nerve cells. Also, very important in keeping the blood and tissue fluids from either becoming too aci or too alkaline, and they allow other nutrients to pass into the blood stream, and aid in transporting nutrients to the cells. They also draw chemicals in and out of the cells, and a slight change in the blood concentration of important minerals can rapidly endanger life. Although the body can manufacture a few vitamins, it can not manufacture a single mineral.

Minerals are also more important to nutrition than vitamins. Vitamins are required for every bodily biochemical process. However, vitamins can not function unless minerals are present. *For example; calcium is needed for vitamin C utilization, zinc is needed fo vitamin "A", magnesium for "B" complex vitamins, and selenium for vitamin "E" absorption, etc.* And according to a US Senate study (Document No.264), 99% of Americans are deficient in **minerals and trace elements.**

Deficiencies In Human Nutrition

The foods average Americans eat, are over processed and void of many essential nutrients, and are grown in soils that have been over planted and saturated with synthetic fertilizers and pesticides. Consequently, Americans are not getting the vitamins and minerals they need in order to stay healthy and ward off diseases, thus their diets must be supplemented with minerals and trace elements. According to The Doctor's Vitamin and Mineral Encyclopedia, *Mineral insufficiency and trace elements insufficiency are more likely to occur than are vitamin insufficiency states.*

Humans must consume vitamins periodically to avoid deficiency and disease. The human body can also store vitamins A, D, and B12 in significant amounts in the liver, in which an adult's diet may be deficient in vitamins A and D for many months and B12 in some cases for years, before developing a deficiency condition. However, vitamin B3 (niacin and niacinamide) is not stored in the human body in significant amounts, so stores may last only a couple of weeks. Deficiencies for vitamins occurs when an organism does not get enough of the vitamins from its food source. For example, in vitamins C (scurvy), in B1(beriberi), in B3(pellagra), and in vitamin D (rickets).

Why Are We Nutritionally Deficient?

The depletion of minerals from our soils has resulted from weather deterioration due to climate changes and major storms washing a way the fertile top soil and other factors such as - over farming, overuse of pesticides, herbicides, and fertilizers. Fruits, vegetables, and grains grown in these soils are becoming mineral deficient. Therefore, w can no longer get sufficient minerals from our food to supply our needs. Experts say that the vast majority of American's are becoming mineral starved!

According to the USDA, in 1953 a person could get all of the vitamin A content he or sh needed from eating 2 peaches. Today, you would have to eat 50 peaches! Many of our foods that are grown for our modern day diet are actually empty of essential nutrients and egin to deplete our body's reserve even faster. Over time this can lead to nutritional eficiencies which may result in loss of energy, less resistance to disease and eventually l health. Vitamin and mineral deficiency is now known to be a more important problem 1an any one imagined. For decades the lack of key vitamins and minerals has been 1own to cause anemia, cretinism, blindness, and goiter that afflict many millions of the vorld's population.

ecent research shows that this is only the tip of a very large iceberg. It is now known 1at even a moderate level of deficiency, with no clinical symptoms, can have devastating onsequences. Affecting perhaps a third of the world's people. Some examples of what as been learned about vitamin/mineral deficiency in the last decade are:

1. It is the world's leading cause of mental impairment, lowering the intellectual capacity of nations.
2. It compromises the immune system, leading to the deaths of over one million children a year with poor health & growth for many more children.
3. It causes an estimated 250,000 serious birth defects every year.
4. It is associated with a significant increase in deaths from heart disease and stroke.
5. Is responsible for the deaths of 60,000 women a year in childbirth.

Vhile the USDA, the FDA, news media and nearly all of "modern medicine" promote accines, chemicals, surgery, and radiation as the accepted way of dealing with the rowing number of illnesses and symptoms prevalent in the US. Various data sources, icluding the US government, suggest that the number of Americans now deficient in 1agnesium is approximately 90%, with some data even suggesting the number to be igher. Iron deficiencies is also estimated at 58%%, folate (folic acid) deficiency is esponsible for over 200,000 severe birth defects every year in several countries, and half f the children with vitamin and mineral deficiencies are in fact suffering from multiple eficiencies, adding up to epidemic proportions.

oday, it is known that these moderate or mild nutritional deficiencies are extremely ommon in almost all countries. The alarming fact is that food now being raised on 1illions of acres of land no longer contain enough minerals, are starving us, no matter ow much we eat. Lacking vitamins, our system can not make the use of minerals, but icking minerals, vitamins are useless -(Senate Document 264, 74th Congress, 1936).

Deficiencies In The US Population
- **Magnesium – 90%**
- **Iron – 58%**
- **Copper - 81%**
- **Manganese – 50%**
- **Chromium – 50%**
- **Zinc - 67%**

hese deficiencies are the result of soil depletion and demineralization that gets worse very so many years due weather and climate change and destruction such as – lack of ain, storms, hurricanes, high temperatures that cause the depletion of minerals. In 1900, orests covered 40% of the earths surface. Today the figure is about 27% (Relating Land

Use and Global land Cover, Turner, 1992).

According to a paper read at the 1994 meeting of the International Society for Systems Sciences, this marks the first time that the "mineral content available to forest and agricultural root systems is down 25 to 40%". Less forest means less top soil. In the pas 200 years the US has lost as much as 75% of its top soil. According to John Robbins in his Pultizer – nominated work Diet for a New America.

Solutions – How To Identify The Signs of Nutrient Deficiency

Informing the public about the need to increase the uptake about the kind of foods that can increase the intake and absorption of vitamins and minerals, and learning how to recognize nutritional deficiencies and imbalance is the key in establishing a healthy nutritional profile. The recommended daily allowance (RDA) that the government has se for vitamins and minerals is the guide many vitamin manufacturers use. It is meant to provide a suggested daily intake of the vitamins and minerals necessary to "prevent" severe nutritional deficiencies in 90% of the population. However, the RDA does not reflect optimal levels of vitamins and minerals, nor does it take into account of varying individual needs for increased amounts of vitamins and minerals during stress, sickness or chronic degenerative conditions.

The chart below explains the signs and symptoms the body gives of nutritional deficiencies before an overt disease develops. This chart is useful for identifying early indications of any nutritional deficiencies that may occur.

Physical Signs of Nutritional Deficiencies
To Common Causes of Mystery Symptoms

Here are some clues to mystery symptoms that often go by undetected from countless trips to the doctors office despite medical testing. Some of these nutritional deficiencies are the more common ones in society today that often go undetected. This chart will help those afflicted with these symptoms that might closely resemble yours. It is sad that mos medical teaching institutions do not focus on nutrition, so many medical professionals ar not equipped to recognize the signs of nutritional deficiencies until you, the patient is extremely sick. The impact of nutritional deficiencies on health should be common knowledge among the medical professional community, but unfortunately, this is not the case!

Vitamin – D > Vitamin D deficiencies are the most common deficiency in the world. Vitamin D is produced naturally in the skin from sun exposure from the ultraviolet rays of the sun. Vitamin D also functions as a steroid hormone in the body, where it can influence the activity of various genes, turning them on or off. Most people who do not get enough vitamin D in their diet today and from lack of sun exposure often experience a wide variety of mystery symptoms that may be difficult to explain. And these symptoms are either short or long term symptoms.

The common short term symptoms of vitamin D are – **Rickets**, caused by a deficiency in vitamin D, calcium, and phosphorus. **Depression**, studies show that vitamin

3 can alleviate seasonal affective disorder during the winter months. **Mood swings, iritability, and fatigue**.

Weakened immune system – can cause **frequent colds & flu**, vitamin d also decreases the chances of developing diseases as multiple sclerosis. **Psoriasis and other skin diseases** are also signs of vitamin d deficiencies.

Long Term symptoms of vitamin D – Osteoporosis; **weak and brittle bones** are common symptoms of deficiencies, where severe cases end with osteoporosis. **Various forms of cancer** have been found with an association of vitamin D deficiency **(breast & prostate cancers)**. **Heart disease,** people with low levels of vitamin D have twice the chance of developing cardiovascular disease – the number one killer, compared to those who had adequate levels.

Conclusion – There are also many other health issues associated with vitamin D deficiency such as – muscle weakness, obesity, high cholesterol, chronic pain cognitive impairment in older individuals, increased risk of bone fractures, diabetes, and many more. People may not even know that they are deficient in vitamin D, since these symptoms may be subtle and perhaps never noticed until old age, when there is an increased chance of developing serious illness. The only way to know if you are deficient or not is to have your doctor do a blood test for a 25(OH) D test done. If your levels are below 30ng/ml then you have a deficiency. If so, increase your sun exposure to just 15 minutes in the early morning or late afternoon is sufficient enough to absorb this very essential nutrient, or taking vitamin D3 as a supplement with 1,000 to 2,000 IU's per day can get your levels back up to normal. **Including foods high in vitamin D** will surely be a better option, and they include – **eggs, herring, cod liver oil, dried shiitake mushrooms, raw button mushrooms, fortified milk, liver, fish oils, and sardines.**

Magnesium deficiency - magnesium deficiency has become a growing health crisis in America today. This unknown mineral is more important than most people think, it is the 4th most abundant mineral in the human body, with 66% of it is found in bone and 33% in skeletal muscle and cardiac muscle. Magnesium is involved in 300 essential biochemical reactions in the body that take affect on a daily basis such as digestion, energy production, muscle function, bone formation, creation of new cells, relaxation of muscles, activation of B vitamins, and the proper functioning of the adrenal glands, kidneys, heart, nervous system and the brain.

Deficiencies in this trace mineral are quite common and can lead to a host of mystery symptoms that are difficult to diagnose. The symptoms of a magnesium deficiency are many and include – **difficulty concentrating, insomnia, anxiety, phobias, irritability, behavioral problems, sensitivity to light and sound, muscle twitching and cramps, trembling, allergies, fatigue, chronic fatigue & fibroblast, and severe pms symptoms.**

Some of the more obvious ones are – **headaches(migraine), high blood pressure, anxiousness, nervousness, re-occurring kidney stones, inability to sleep, irritability, abnormal heart rhythm, and muscle tension and cramps.**

The importance of this mineral can not be over stated, and as far back as 1971, that

Dr. Edmund B. Fink (a magnesium expert and researcher at the University of West Virginia School of Medicine in Morgantown), recorded in the "The Executive Health" that:

- **Magnesium deficiency not only exists but is common**
- **Although its common, it is often undetected**
- **Chronic deficiencies can produce long-term damage and can be fatal**
- **The manifestations of the deficiency are many and varied**

Conclusion: Deficiencies in this mineral are quite common and it is estimated that 80 to 90% of the population may be deficient in this very important mineral. If you suffer from mental illness, muscle pain or disorders, or have any of the above symptoms, you may be deficient in magnesium. A hair mineral analysis test may be a great way of determining your levels of magnesium along with any other nutrients.

Foods rich in magnesium include – dark green leafy vegetables, beans, legumes, buckwheat, almonds, cashews, pine nuts, halibut, chocolate, whole grains, tofu, and potatoes. Also taking magnesium supplements with a balanced diet comprising of seafood, nuts, whole grains, dark green leafy vegetables can go along way in restoring your magnesium levels back to normal. Foods rich in magnesium are also heat sensitive, and cooking voids the potency of magnesium, so steaming your vegetables or eating more salads can be quite helpful in maintaining optimal levels in your blood stream.

Iron deficiency – iron deficiency often causes iron-deficient anemia. Every red blood cell in the body contains iron in its hemoglobin, the pigment that carries oxygen to the tissues from the lungs. Those with this deficiency often will experience the following **symptoms – extreme fatigue, dizziness upon standing up, headaches, poor circulation, pale skin, gums, and ridges on nails, mouth sores & fissures at corners of the mouth, tingling in the extremities, brain fog, and stomach disorders – heart burn, flatulence, & abdominal pain.** Iron deficiency anemia (IDA), often caused by insufficient iron intake, is the major cause of anemia in childhood.

Some of the causes of IDA include – insufficient iron in the diet, poor absorption by the body, ongoing blood loss, mostly from menstruation, and periods of rapid growth in children.

Those who are at risk the most are vegetarians, and women with heavy periods or women who use (IUD's) to prevent pregnancies are more at risk for developing iron deficiency. In extreme cases of iron deficiency, anemia can lead to the need of blood transfusions. Supplementing your diet with whole food iron supplements should be enough for most people, however a variety of foods can provide you with **great sources of iron – lean meats, egg yolks, spinach, green leafy vegetables, dried beans, blackstrap molasses, raisins, and whole wheat.**

Conclusion: Proper nutritional intake, which includes a diet rich in iron, is most important for all people, especially children. Establishing good eating habits will help prevent iron deficiency and iron deficient anemia.

Vitamin K – Vitamin k helps the body coagulate blood properly. Vitamin k is essential or healthy dense bones. Its deficiency often shows up in bone related problems like loss f bone (osteopenia), decrease in bone mineral density (osteoporosis), and fractures ncluding hip fractures. **The following signs of a vitamin K deficiency are** – **most ommon is heavy menstrual bleeding; gum bleeding, nose bleeds that don't stop, blood in the urine & stools, calcification of heart valves, prolonged clotting times, anemia, and easy bruising.**

Deficiencies of vitamin k can be prevented by consuming and appropriate **diet consisting f green leafy vegetables, collard greens, spinach, turnips, eggs, and soybeans.**

Conclusion: If you feel you may have a vitamin k deficiency, supplement with 65mgs of vitamin K for women and 80mgs for men. Prescriptions of vitamin k from doctors often depends upon the severity of the condition of the individual as a oral medicine for a certain period of time.

Omega 3 Fatty Acids – Omega 3 fatty acid is an essential fatty acid, meaning the body can not produce it on it's own, and its sources must come from food. This is a common deficiency problem in which there are many associated mystery symptoms associated with it, and they **include – fatigue, poor skin condition, psoriasis, dry brittle hair & nails, creaking and popping joints, bowel disorders (IBS& Crohn's), high blood pressure, heart disease, diabetes, depression, ADHD & learning disorders, mood disorders and behavioral problems.**

In an ideal world, we would normally get enough of omega 3 we needed from fish. Unfortunately, most of the world's waters are contaminated with mercury and other harmful substances. Many people are now beginning to add fish oils to their diet, but make sure your fish oil is organic krill oil and purchase no more than 60 gel caps at a time for their optimum omega 3 supplementation, as buying it in bulk can go rancid before you finish half of the bottle.

Conclusion: Omega 3 deficiency is becoming quite common and is considered one of the important nutrients for optimal and necessary health. Make sure you include in your diet natural sources of omega 3's like – flax seeds, nuts and seeds, eggs, lean meats, walnuts, almond and almond butter, oats, beans, wheat germ, and wheat bran are all good sources.

Niacin – A niacin deficiency or B3 can also cause strange symptoms. The most common being are – **fatigue & muscle weakness, depression, canker sores, loss of appetite, dizziness, headaches, and mental disturbances**. A severe form of niacin deficiency is called "pellagra" and those with pellagra exhibit the following symptoms – red swollen tongue, dry carcked skin, severe diarrhea, and dementia.

Niacin can be found in dietary sources of poultry, dairy products, eggs, milk, green vegetables, beans, and red meats. Those with severe niacin deficiency may benefit by taking supplements of B3. It is also to remember that taking niacin may cause a flushing effect that is virtually harmless and goes a way within 15 minutes or so. Start off with a low dose and increase it slowly.

Zinc – This is one of the most essential minerals to the body because it is responsible for regulating normal enzymatic functions throughout the body. **Those who may have a zinc deficiency will often exhibit the following symptoms – menstrual irrigulaqrites fertility problems & loss of libido, difficulty in sleeping, loss of smell, hair loss and dandruff, white spots on nails, nail cuticle inflammation, bowel disease, skin conditions – dry skin, eczema, psoriasis, low sperm count in men, low testosterone levels, and acne.**

If you believe that you have a zinc deficiency that may be causing your mystery symptoms, **increase your consumption of foods such as oysters, meats, poultry, nuts pumpkin seeds, eggs and whole wheat products. Supplements of zinc are also useful and it is not beneficial to take in more than 50mgs of zinc, anything over 100mgs can weaken your immune system.**

Potassium – This mineral is very important for the proper functioning of – heart beat, muscles, nervous system, and the circulatory system. Low potassium levels or (**Hypokalemia**) has a number of symptoms associated with it, **including – fatigue, muscle weakness, cramps, dry skin, unexplained chills, unquenchable thirst, irregular heart rhythm, insomnia, irritability, anxiety, mental confusion, glucose intolerance, diarrhea, nausea, and vomiting.**

High cholesterol is also a sign of low potassium levels, although it can also be caused by other factors as well. In extreme deficiencies it can lead to cardiac arrest. Excess use of diuretics, fasting, laxatives can lead to deficiency states. Alcoholics are also at a risk for this and other important vitamins and minerals.

To increase your potassium levels through the use of foods are the best way, and they include – **baked potatoes, raisins, lima beans, grapes, oranges, apricots, bananas, dates, figs, tomatoes, and spinach.**

Conclusion – There can be many causes of deficiency for potassium and that can be from poor health and diet, illness, body being unable to absorb potassium, eating disorders (bulimia), and the use of medications.
Learn to judge by the signs and symptoms of this very important mineral and do yourself good by including it in your diet and through regular supplementation, be careful in not over dosing with potassium as it can also lead to health problems. Following the required potassium intake prescribed from the manufactures is fine and well, provide caution in not over doing it!

Folic Acid – A folic acid deficiency "anemia" happens when your body does not get enough folic acid in your diet. Folic acid is one of the important B vitamins that help your body make new cells, including red blood cells in which your body needs red blood cells to carry oxygen. And it is also needed for DNA synthesis, DNA repair, and a healthy functioning of the entire body. If you don't have enough of red blood cells, you'll have anemia, which can make you feel very tired and weak. Some people just don't get enough of this vital nutrient from their diet on a daily basis or have trouble absorbing it from the foods they eat. Pregnant women who do not get enough of folic acid often have serious birth defects. Folic acid also works with vitamins B12 and iron to help form new blood cells of the body.

The most common symptoms and signs are – weakness, fatigue and lethargy, mouth redness and sores, pale skin and gums, depression, gray hair, and hyperpigmentation.

Symptoms of folic acid include – feeling weak & tired, often feeling light headed, being forgetful, being grouchy, loss of appetite, trouble concentrating, mood swings, pallor (unusually pale skin), shortness of breath with exertion, sore smooth tongue, poor balance, cracked lips at corners of your mouth, poor balance, and chest pain & irregular heart beat.

Severe deficiency leads to anemia).

Mental behavior symptoms include – difficult learning, paranoia, psychosis, mood swings, and mania.
Most people with a folic acid deficiency must take supplements to correct it. And most people who suffer from heart burn often take anti-acids, which can prevent the absorption of folic acid. Instead of taking anti-acids try hydrochloric acid supplements.

Causes of deficiency can be caused by – diseases in which folic acid is not absorbed well, such as "Celiac" disease or "Crohn's" disease, drinking excess alcohol, eating over cooked foods, medications such as dilantin, sulfasalazine, or trimethoprim-sulfamethoxazole, and poor diet which is often seen in the elderly and people who do not eat fresh fruits or vegetables.

Conclusion – The importance of Folic acid is of an extreme, folic acid is critical in normal pregnancies in helping to prevent birth defects, such as **"spinal bifida"** and other related diseases. These can be major birth defects that can usually happen within the first few weeks of pregnancies, before a women even knows that she is pregnant. Foods rich in folic acid are – beans, legumes, citrus fruits, dark green leafy vegetables, liver, poultry, pork, wheat bran, and other whole grains.

Chromium – A very important essential mineral that's becoming of an epidemic in the US. It is one of the key minerals involved in blood sugar metabolism and fat levels of the body. As the main component of glucose tolerance factor (GTF), chromium assists insulin in reducing blood sugar by stimulating glucose uptake by the muscles and other tissues. The functions of chromium are – regulates blood sugar, moderates cholesterol levels, promotes arterial health, boosts the immune system, and stimulates protein synthesis.

The short term deficiency symptoms of chromium are – hypo & hyper-glycemia, diabetes, fatigue, arterial disease, obesity, high cholesterol, and mood swings. Factors that reduce chromium levels are – diets that are high in refined carbohydrates, such as white flour products, white pasta, white rice, potatoes, and processed foods, all will use up chromium at a high rate which can lead to deficiencies.
Most common signs are – fatigue, blood sugar imbalance, mood swings, high cholesterol, and obesity.

Conclusion – It has been suggested that a minimum of 200mcgs per day should be

used by non-diabetic adults. People that generally require chromium are those who are overweight, people who eat high carbohydrates, and people who do very little exercise.

If you have been suffering from a mystery symptoms for a long while and one or more of the above vitamin and mineral deficiencies seem to apply to you, begin by adding supplements to your diet. Sometimes it's a little harder to get the nutrients needs from the foods we eat since environmental toxins and pollution makes soil much more depleted than it was a 100 years ago. Adding whole food supplements to your diet may be all that you need to solve your mystery symptoms and learn to live the healthy life you so deserve.

Don't give up and listen to your body's cries for help and learn to recognize the signs and symptoms that it is trying to tell you. No matter what you've heard from doctors, friends, co-workers, and family, you're not crazy and its not all in your head, or maybe it is all in your head
exactly! Always listen in what the body tells you, with a little patients and by learning to recognizing the symptoms, you can then prevent ill health and disease and save yourself from a trip to the emergency room and hospital!

BODY LANGUAGE OF LOVE SIGNALS

Did you ever wish there was a way or method of knowing the common body signals of love and attraction? Or wondering if he or she is attracted to you? Well, there is way, and science has studied this sort of behavior and can tell you what these signals mean, or how you can tell or read the body signals of the opposite sex. Here's how men and women can learn to master the art of love.

For ever unconscious movement, there's a bodily reaction or signal if you may. Body language is hard wired to our brain and the body unconsciously reacts. Regardless of what sex you may be, if you want to learn how to recognize these non-verbal signals and increase your chances in the matting game, then you should see below and learn how to decode gestures of attraction and mating.

Signals Of Attraction Men Need To Decode From Women

When women toss or flick their hair – while talking to you, it definitely means she's interested in you. If she's looking at some one else while talking to you, well, better luck next time.

When women fiddle or play with round objects – or fondling a phallic-shaped such as the stem of a wine glass or a dangling earring while giving you repeated glances, means she is finds you attractive, and is approachable.

When a women unconsciously touches herself – A women that is slowly touching or caressing herself on the neck, throat, or thigh. Means if a man plays his cards right, he too may get to touch in the same way. This is the body's language at the most basic level.

When women point their knees – sitting with one leg tucked up under her, chances are at the knee pointing outwards is pointing towards the person she finds most interesting. opefully that is you!

When a women put their face on display – women who are trying to attract a man's tention, will often rest their elbows on a flat surface top, and place one hand on top of e other, then place her chin on her hands and face directly to him as if she is offering it him for admiration. It also indicates that **the man has her full attention, and is open flattery and advances.**

Signals of Attraction Women Need To Decode

len normally don't play the courtship game as women do, they only respond to it. But ey also, have their comparative measures as well. Here are some tips for women when ur eye's meet his.

When men have protruding thumbs – In many hand gestures that men portray, they present strength of character and the ego. A man will often use his protruding thumbs, front of his pockets, around women to whom he is attracted too.

When men display their crotch – most women already know this, when men sit with eir legs spread wide at her, as if he was taking a picture. This is called the crotch isplay showing his masculinity, letting who ever is observing know that he isn't going 1ywhere.

When men try hard – To make themselves more appealing, men will unconsciously range their clothing by straightening their tie, collars, adjust their trousers and brush the naginary dust off their shoulders, he's telling you indirectly that he wants to look the ery best for you.

When men take up space – They often do this by trying to occupy as much space as ossible to become more noticeable. He may also start to rock back and forth on the soles f his feet as if he was making love in a standing position.

When their fingers point to what he wants you to notice – When a man tucks his 1umbs into his belt or into the tops of the pockets to frame the genital area, it indicates a exually aggressive attitude. This gesture shows a women he is ready for action, nwillingly giving away what's really on his mind.

Body Language Tips For Men

Vhen women slowly cross and uncrosses their legs, then this means she is into you.

Vhen women put their handbag close to you, it means they like you! If not her legs ould stay firmly in place.

a women puts her handbag close to you, it means she likes you! But if she has it lutched around her arms, watch out !!

Vhen women have their legs together and body facing away from you, you are going home alone!

Body Language Tips For Women

When a man puts his hands in his pockets, it means he's closed off and not interested.

When a man mirrors a women's facial expressions, she'll think he is caring and attractive

When a man is wearing tight-fitting trousers, small-size speedos or dangling the long en of a belt or a bunch of keys in front of his crotch, it means he's putting his masculinity o display. The same thing as if a women wearing a push up bra.

Common Gestures of Boredom

- Jiggling feet is a sign of boredom.

- Locked ankles show negative emotions.

- Extended blinking, covering of the mouth, rubbing the eyes all mean the person is lying.

For those of you interested in learning more of body signals of love and attraction, read Allan Pease - "The Body Language of Love".

www.ingramcontent.com/pod-product-compliance
Lightning Source LLC
Chambersburg PA
CBHW070459290526
45790CB00003B/1013

* 9 7 8 1 4 8 1 8 5 2 9 0 6 *